Hair

Public, Political,
Extremely Personal

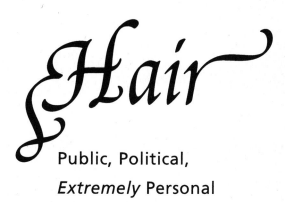

Hair

Public, Political,
Extremely Personal

Diane Simon

THOMAS DUNNE BOOKS
St. Martin's Griffin
New York

THOMAS DUNNE BOOKS
An imprint of St. Martin's Press

www.stmartins.com

Library of Congress Cataloging-in-Publication Data
Simon, Diane.
    Hair : public, political, extremely personal / Diane Simon
        p. cm.
    Includes bibliographical references.
    ISBN 0-312-20893-6 (hc)
    ISBN 0-312-27851-9 (pbk)
    1. Hair—Social aspects. 2. Fashion—United States. I. Title
GT2295.U5 S56 2000
391.5—dc21   99-089749

First St. Martin's Griffin Edition: July 2001

10 9 8 7 6 5 4 3 2 1

To my mother, Wilma Simon,
and in memory of my father, Robert Simon

Contents

Acknowledgments

I owe a great many thanks:

First to those brave souls who became the subjects of these chapters, for sharing their hair with a stranger.

To my agent, Jane Dystel, and her associate, Miriam Goderich, and to my editor, Melissa Jacobs, for showing faith in that which did not yet exist.

To my excellent readers—Laura Brahm, Jane Murgo, Benny Ogorek, Hilary Rao, and Jeff Sharlet—for making this a better book.

To Catherine Allgor, Richard Condon, Steven Cramer, Ann Kahn, Sue Leonard, David Leubke, Jen Nessel, Kathy Peiss, Richard Sandomir, Bob Tamarkin, Graham White, and Shane White, for lending their work, their expertise, and their acquaintances.

To my colleagues and students at Ramaz, for giving me something else to think about.

To David Waldstreicher, who gave me a push.

To my family—Paul and Chantal Goldblum, Wilma Simon, Victoria Simon, Jane Simon—for always knowing the difference between what's funny and what's for dinner. Special thanks go to Jane, whose hair acts like mine, and to Victoria, whose hair does not. I'm sorry that Judith Simon and Margaret Smith, who did not live to see this completed, will not see their names here; I don't know if I thanked them enough.

For always being where I could find them, to Scott Cole, Mark Goble, Doc and Bibs Pankin, Teri Pankin Schobinger, Elisa Tamarkin, and Liz Tingley.

And especially to Benny Ogorek, who drove me to Borough Park and picked me up, and whose wisdom always makes a difference. He is a privilege.

Finally, to my straight-haired mother, Wilma Simon, who makes everything possible. She might not feel the pain of her kinky-haired daughters, but she is generous, patient, and deserving of much more than even these deeply felt thanks. Everything good here is for her.

The Haircut

At thirteen what I hated most
Was not the aftermath of slicked-
Down stickiness, nor the barber's
Wet breath misting on my ear,
The sting as his scissors
Nipped cartilage or lobe;
And not the fuming barbicides
In formation like Prohibition
Booze, the faced-off mirrors
Doubling the damage done
To duck's ass, Beatle bangs,
Curlicues descending from
The temples to dissemble
As sideburns . . .

     With a hiss
My mother buzzed her palm
From nape to crown, following
Her orders to spot-check
Each half inch cropped.
Drafted to cast her lot
Against my flowering anima,
She watched my bristling
Scalp as I glowered home,
Placing a city block between us,
Sweating to outgrow that skirt-
Clinging youngest son
Undone without his camouflage.

Even after the glancing
Jolt of the shop windows,
My head unbearably shrunken,
As if I'd held my nose, ears,
And mouth and sucked in hard;
Even after I showered off
The fallout and blow-dried

The stubble nibbling my neck,
The worst came down at dinner
In the weight of Father's hand
Kneading my bare shoulders,
And my home-grown estrangements
Clipped to a truth I hated to admit:
Shorn like that it *was* a shock
How much we looked alike.

—Steven Cramer

Hair

Public, Political,
Extremely Personal

One

Kinky Living in a Straight World
A Prelude to Hair

Before you go to school, it probably doesn't matter. Even if it hurts when your parents comb it, or it gets long enough to be cut by a woman in a black smock who douses your head with a spray bottle before she snips off your bangs. Even when it is matted with gum or tar from the neighbor's driveway, and a whole hunk of it has to go, I don't think your hair matters to you until you see yourself in the mirror of your friend's eyes. That's when the trouble begins.

I remember being the only one with frizzy curls in a class of twenty sleek-haired girls. It is a memory that could be true of any of my years in school, though of course I remember times when it mattered more than others. I don't think it was important in kindergarten until the very end, when a yearbook picture of my class winding down the hall in a line shows me fourth in line. Though I was tall then, you can't see my face. But your eye is drawn immediately to the back-lit puff of my hair, riding high near the front. In fourth grade it was important again. Mrs. Cox made silhouette tracings of our profiles, cut them out of black construction paper, and made us guess whose was whose. Later, we would label them to hang in the hall. As soon as I understood the project, I knew it would cause me trouble, and I tried to postpone my turn in the portrait seat, hoping that somehow Mrs. Cox would understand and let me off the hook. Of course, she didn't; and of course, everyone guessed my profile first, because it was the only one topped with bumps and ridges. What I wanted most then, and probably still want today, was a ponytail silhouette—a neat facial profile backed by a separate knot of smooth, swingy hair.

The years blend together in my memory, and trends emerge because moments repeat over and over, as if my hair history were a scratched record stuck on a lame refrain. A friend's father asked if he could scrub the family pans with my head. A classmate wondered if she could touch my hair, and I consented against my better judgement. "Oh," she said, drawing her hand away immediately, "it's like hay." Another was surprised that it was soft, since it didn't look it. Most people don't ask before they reach. I've learned to sense the approach of an unwelcome hand and to duck efficiently. Lately, I've added an admonition. "This is not a petting zoo," I say sternly. A few people persist, and I shoot them with a gun I carry just for these emergencies—once in the heart, and again in the head, execution style. I tolerate the people who've told me, over and over, how lucky I am, and that people pay good money to get hair like mine; I tolerate them, but I hate them all the same.

Wild and bristly, my hair has drawn me out of the soft circle of smooth-haired girls and left me on the margins, an onlooker with a kink in her curl. It's not that I tried to rebel—indeed, I longed to conform—but my hair made it impossible. If only there had been a way to subdue it, to force it to adopt a manageable shape and a palatable texture, then I know I would have gone along, but there never was. I shaved it close in patterns, grew it long, and dyed it black, then red, then blond. Twice, I sat still for hours while a Liberian woman braided it and strung it with black and purple beads. It held for weeks and clacked a rhythm when I walked, and I thought for a while I could be black and have braids instead of being Jewish and having frizz. But it didn't hold forever, and I had to return to myself. I'm a stranger in the straight-hair world.

I spent hours combing the midback hair of Midge, an otherwise unremarkable baby-sitter. When I played house with my straight-haired friends, I draped the hood of a brown sweatshirt over my head and pretended what hung down my back was actually a thick, long curtain of hair. If I didn't look in the mirror or touch the stretchy cotton and I ignored the flap of the metal zipper, I could almost convince myself: ah, this is what it's like, heavy and warm. But it wasn't, so I've become an expert in cosmetic strategy. I tote hats stowed in giant flowered hatboxes across the country for humid summer weddings and can tie a turban fast and tight. Sikh cab drivers stop and wave, while others look at me pityingly, wondering if I've been stricken with cancer. If a hairdresser uses the word *coarse* at anytime during our time together, I skip the tip and don't return. But the straight-hair world is not as shiny and smooth as I had imagined; bigger issues than texture loom large on the horizon.

Over time, I've become consultant and confessor, the five-minute hair therapist who knows what it's like to have low hair esteem. A man whose dog plays every morning with my dog wants to know if I think he'll bald from front to back or back to front; one is all right with him, the other isn't. After I placed an ad soliciting stories for this book, my phone rang at three one morning. A young man with a strong Brooklyn accent apologized for waking me; he'd thought that he was calling an office and would get a machine. Wasn't I some type of doctor, maybe a miracle worker or a shaman, he wondered, and was disappointed when I told him I was writing a book. "So, you can't make hair come back?" he asked. "No," I told him. "Would you like to talk about it?" Things change, slowly, imperceptibly. In order to be apart from something, you must in some way be a part of it. It's not that my hair has smoothed out any, or that I've suddenly rediscovered a deeply buried ethnic pride—I haven't. It's just that I've noticed a subtle shift in perspective, which might be explained as adulthood but which is no less troubling for the explanation.

The other day, I was shopping in Albany, New York, with my mother and I saw a little girl, about five, with springy blond curls that stood out all over her head. Her mother was in a dressing room and she was playing with some cards on the floor nearby. She didn't look at me, but I squatted next to her anyway. "Hi," I said. "I like your hair." She continued to play with her cards and ignored me. "Do you hate it? I hated my hair when I was your age," I told her, imagining that I was telling her something that would serve her well. And then, before she had a chance to look up or duck away, I reached over and touched a curl, stretched it between my fingers and let it bounce back. Instantly, without even looking up, she pulled a gun that looked just like mine—shiny and full of purpose. But she was young and too small to hold it properly, so her first shot missed my heart and grazed my arm, her second went wild and hit the wall. I tried to tell myself I'd learned my lesson, I would never do it again, but now I'm not so sure. She really had fabulous hair. People pay a fortune to get hair like that.

Two

Down=to=There Hair
A Brief History of Hair Crisis in America

There were rumors. There were stories. Everything was unmentionable but nothing was unimaginable.

—Joan Didion, *The White Album*

It may have been spawned in the aggressively complacent fifties, the decade Tom Hayden once called the "unpredictable meantime," but America's bouffant came of age in the chaos of the sixties. In 1962, *Newsweek* reported that "among United States teenagers, bouffants are proliferating as fast as the toadstools they resemble." One Chicago teacher estimated that seventy percent of her female students styled their hair into bouffants, and another educator complained—just as eighteenth-century critics had denounced the bouffant's *ancienne cousine*—that some girls were having trouble steering their hair through low and narrow doorways. Few women naturally grew the masses of hair the bouffant required, and that year, the U.S. Department of Commerce noticed that hair imports had gone up over one hundred thousand dollars since 1961. By 1964, the possibilities seemed endless. Salons began to feature false eyelashes, made of human hair, mink, and—for eighty dollars a pair—sable, and to employ specialists, known as *falseticians* to tend to them. The Indian government began gathering from its temples the huge piles of hair sacrificed each week to Lord Venkateswara, producing forty-eight thousand wigs in six months. United States wig sales rose one thousand percent between 1959 and 1967, when they earned an estimated five hundred million dollars a year.

To the counterculture of the late sixties, the bouffant embodied everything that was wrong with America. A shiny, smooth helmet of hair, sprayed immobile and stiff, it neither swayed in the wind nor yielded to the touch. It took a certain amount of hard work to build up, but then modern technology—hair spray, hair dryers—made it relatively easy to maintain; the bouffant would retain its shape until something bigger and stronger pushed it aside. It was, in this way, a uniquely American product, a combination of Yankee ingenuity and perseverance, tough and staunch. But like America in the fifties, the character of the bouffant relied on the reflected light of its own surface. Sometimes, as the decade's burgeoning wig industry attested, the bouffant itself was a false front, a properly toned lamination that streamed from a strategically placed comb. Like a party smile or a government statement, it was a nicety that need not correspond to organic reality. In the proper light, a bouffant might resemble the destructive cloud of the atomic bomb, perhaps necessary but definitely evil. Most important, the bouffant had something to hide: underneath its lacquered veneer swam a tangled mess of knotted hair.

There may not have been one single youth movement in America by the end of the sixties, but one thing the peace-loving hippies shared with the Black Panther militants and the inexhaustible yippies and the secretive, violent Weathermen was an avowed disgust with American hypocrisy, the glossy sheen of domestic bliss and democratic promise that hid our darkest secrets. In the midst of American prosperity, the counterculture saw rampant poverty. Behind a veil of democratic rhetoric, they saw a greedy government using defenseless youths to fight an imperialistic, unwinable war in a faraway land. The central institutions of American life—school, government, and family—seemed corrupt, conspiring as they did to conceal their own dishonesty and to regulate the knowledge and behavior of others to protect the status quo. The counterculture—earnest, wily, angry, and dissolute—prized depth over surface, and imagined themselves the keepers of American "truth." Hypocrisy, writes historian James Farrell, was the "cardinal sin" of the sixties.

This distrust of convention and regulation permeated the counterculture's worldview, linking global politics to personal appearance. If schools, the military, and the government required short hair for men, long for women, it was because of an outdated system of social control, an assertion of gendered assumptions that had everything to do with market capitalism and nothing to do with individual fulfillment and social honesty. Like the military, corporations required masculine prowess, and thus stipulated haircuts that would project authority and discipline. Black Panthers and others who believed in the promise of an alternative beauty rejected the flattened lines of the masculine conk and the feminine hot comb. Instead, they cultivated a defiant round globe of hair that crossed nationalism and religion: it was called an Afro but resembled a halo and seemed to offer its wearers a special transcendence that went beyond added height. Hippie hair, on the other hand, took its political weight from nature and the force of gravity: it was long, unkempt, "down-to-there hair," the kind they celebrated in the eponymous musical. It was hair that seemed to be a harbinger of harmony between body, soul, and society.

This was, after all, a very *physical* movement; in the late 1960s, much of the fight was about actual bodies—how they were handled, clothed, used, and, finally, destroyed. The hippie movement worked to dispel the cloud of shame that had settled on America's bedrooms by declaring sex essential, liberating, and fun. Timothy Leary pronounced hedonism America's new religion, and the Sexual Freedom League touted honesty, simplicity, and the intangible necessity of Eros. *Time* magazine summed up the Summer of Love with a "Hippie Code," rules for a life without rules: "Do your own thing, wherever you have to do it and whenever you want. Drop out. Leave society as you have known it. Leave it utterly. Blow the mind of every straight person you can reach. Turn them on, if not to drugs, then to beauty, love, honesty, and fun." In this world, getting stoned, growing your hair, and celebrating your nudity in public were political acts, revolutionary assaults on a corrupt regime.

Hence, the utter perfection of *Hair,* which tunneled through the rhetoric and confusion to come up with a single striking emblem. Immensely successful, the show opened on April 19, 1969—a date chosen by the show's astrologer, Maria Elise Crummaire—and closed 1,750 performances and twenty-two million dollars gross later. Galt MacDermot's score sets the cries of hippie protest—against Vietnam, against racism, and poverty—to the tribal rhythms of the Bantus, creating an anthem for a generation. Long, wild, and triumphantly coifed, the hair of *Hair* became a banner for the hippie message, an updated melange of sentiment, patriotism, and religious ecstasy:

Let it fly in the breeze
and get caught in the trees
give a home to the bees
in my hair! . . . Oh say can you see . . . my eyes?
If you can, then my hair's too short . . . My hair like Jesus wore it
Alleluia, I adore it!

When, in the opening scene, the gang sacrifices a lock of Claude's hair, the audience witnesses a solemn act of tribal propitiation, but also the solidification of a cultural metaphor: Claude's hair burns and crinkles like a draft card; later, his body will succumb to the fire of enemy guns.

A quick perusal of popular media shows that *Hair* did not manufacture the zeitgeist; it reflected it. During the years of *Hair*'s peak popularity, the *New York Times Index* records reference after reference to hair conflicts and controversies. Personal appearance was an essential element of social order for both sides of the struggle, especially where young men were concerned. Long hair seemed to indicate a latent femininity, a premonition especially dangerous for a country that relied on its men for both military courage and market instinct. Long-haired men were denied unemployment benefits in Monterey, California, because officials reasoned that they had voluntarily rendered themselves unemployable, as had women who wore microminis. (In a rare moment of barely concealed hilarity, the *New York Times* records a comment by Monterey lawyer Francis Heisler, who was particularly incensed by the miniskirt ruling. He insisted that this type of rule should be "stopped before it spreads.")

In 1970, a federal court in Boston ordered schools to reinstate students suspended for wearing long hair, but a Savannah federal court sided with the school board against a long-haired student. The only merit scholar at one Pennsylvania school attended class from home via a telephone hookup, because though the courts had supported his right to wear his hair long and receive his education, the school principal could not abide a fashion he considered a grave disruption. A year later, Supreme Court Justice Hugo Black, who the *Times* reports was then "all but bald and going on 85," elaborated on the Court's decision not to consider a case brought by Chesley Carr, a Texas high school student who asked that the courts strike down his school's no-long-hair policy pending a decision by a lower Texas court. Justice Black noted that the Constitution does not "give high school boys the right to wear their hair long." At the same time, the *Times* reports, "Justice Black said on Thursday lawyers should not be pressing the Supreme Court with 'emergency motions,' implying that the nation will be in crisis unless long hair is allowed."

And yet, the nation *was* in crisis: a fifteen-year-old boy was scalped in May of 1970 by self-proclaimed patriot vigilantes, who saw his long hair as un-American. Hundreds of school boards confronted thousands of students who defied traditional standards of decent dress. Billboards all across the country urged young people to do their part for their country: "Beautify America," they said, "Get a Haircut." At the Redwood High School in suburban San Francisco, the athletic director, Robert J. Troppman, resigned his post when the school's superintendent temporarily suspended the school's policy against long hair for athletes. Troppmen told the *Times*, "I think this is the beginning of the end of all athletics. . . . There are things like uniformity and discipline involved." A federal judge later upheld the school's preexisting policy, ruling against the long-haired athletes. "In these perilous, troubled times," wrote the judge, "when discipline in certain quarters appears to be an ugly word, it should not be considered unreasonable nor regarded as an impingement of constitutional prerogatives to require plaintiffs to bring themselves within the spirit, purpose, and intendments of the questioned rule." Short hair, in San Francisco at least, was good medicine.

Other countries were also affected by the paroxysms of the American youth movement. The mayor of San Miguel de Allende ordered police to crop the hair of all long-haired men found in the town center, and a newly renovated post office in Singapore was decorated with posters reminding patrons of the ugliness of long-haired men. On an aggressive campaign against "dishonest elements," including ruffians, gamblers, opium smokers, and prostitutes, the South Vietnamese police used bayonets to cut the hair of over a thousand young men, whose hair was said to violate the "good customs and morals of our country." In recognition of the distinction between morals and morale, however, the Vietnamese government issued long-hair permits to certain rock performers. Ding Bui of the Firestones received permission to "have long hair and wear special clothes for the years 1970 and 1971." But according to the *New York Times*, another group, the New Flintstone Corporation, was shorn without mercy by the police.

When Richard Corson, preeminent hair historian, described the bouffant of the fifties at the tail end of the hair turmoil of the sixties, he could only do it in terms of generational conflict, making the bouffant a parable for the hair wars of a new era. Teachers hated it, he noticed, since it seemed to distract their students. Visually, it was imposing, keeping some from seeing the blackboard, and hygienically, it was a disaster, requiring enough hair spray to hold for weeks at a time. One girl, in Canton, Ohio, had left her bouffant for so long that a colony of roaches had taken up residence inside. She hadn't felt any disturbance, but a classmate noticed blood on the girl's neck. The image is Corson's implied narrative of transition from the fifties to the sixties: a peaceful shell had shattered and the roaches were scurrying for cover. The consensus that the nation had imagined, forged in the aftermath of World War II, unraveled as the Cold War continued and America's involvement in Vietnam escalated without results.

The threat of encroaching communists could only be a shadow; it was clear that for the United States, the enemy came from within.

The only absolute seemed to be an increasing dissonance, a dislocation between expectation, truth, and reality. Order seemed a thing of the past, a quality lamented and pined after but rarely achieved. More Americans than ever before attended college in the 1960s, yet increasingly visible thousands were choosing to become dropouts, rejecting the conventional fruits of social conformity. Five days after the signing of landmark civil rights legislation, the Watts section of Los Angeles exploded in violence. Thirty-four were dead, countless injured, four thousand arrested. Abbie Hoffman and Jerry Rubin threw dollar bills onto the floor of the New York Stock Exchange from a balcony above and gleefully declared "money is over." Even *Hair*, which prided itself on "frankness" and adopted a stage design that exposed the inner workings of a Broadway production with visible scaffolding, stage crews, and open cues, was actually a case in point—a careful rehearsal of controlled spontaneity.

Early in the fifties, the CIA had experimented with LSD, hoping to use it as a truth serum for captive enemy spies. Even when that possibility was abandoned, agents continued taking the drug, hoping to learn to maintain composure should an enemy slip some into their drinks. A 1954 memo forbade the use of LSD as an ingredient in CIA Christmas party punches. This was just a foreshadowing of the trouble to come. Like the use of LSD, the very notion of "truth" in America had slipped from the bounds of administrative control. While the counterculture assailed hypocrisy in every form, and disciplinarians thundered on about order, a *Fortune* editorialist worried that in the case of America's angry youth, rhetoric and reality might indeed be one and the same. "These youngsters are acting out a revolution," the writer warned. "This is what they say they are doing . . . and this is what they *are* doing." But when the *New York Times* asked Spiro Agnew if his lengthening sideburns meant that the Nixon administration was trying to change course and appeal to American youth, Agnew replied, "No . . . It's just an effort on my part to make my photographs make me look as though I'm not bald from halfway up. The gray hair doesn't show in the pictures."

Their faces were as the faces of men; and they had hair as the hair of women.

—Nicholas Noyes, "An Essay Against Periwigs"

Of course, America's hair crisis of the 1960s was not unique. Ever since Caesar insisted on shaving the heads of the newly conquered Gauls and turning their unattached blond hair into wigs of victory, ever since the Emperor Tertullian warned his people that wigs were the "inventions of the devil," and might lead to damnation, hair has been a subject of public controversy. For centuries, it has earned the combined attentions of religious and political leaders. In the Judeo-Christian world, where social order is often associated with religious rectitude, politicians and preachers alike have considered Paul's first letter to the Corinthians a divine guide to righteous hair. "Does not nature itself teach you," Paul asked, "that for a man to wear long hair is degrading to him, but if a woman wears long hair it is her pride?" Long, suitably hidden hair became, for women, a sign of faith in God and hence, a sign of assumed social responsibility; for men, it was short hair. Though throughout the Christian world there were certainly long periods of time when men wore long hair and Paul's fashion directive fell into disuse, his distinctions were never erased from the collective memory of Christian consciousness; they represented a structured ideal in which gender distinctions formed the underpinnings of a well-ordered, godly society. Paul and his Corinthian followers haunt every era of hair crisis in the Western world.

The ghost of Paul probably arrived in America aboard the *Mayflower*, since the Virginia settlers were not as conscientious a group as the Puritans of Plymouth. In England, the conflict between Cavaliers and Puritans that propelled New England's settlers would lead to the beheading of one king and, finally, the importation of another. In New England, it provided a spiritual lodestar, a guide for the erection of God's kingdom in the wilderness. Ostensibly a challenge to England's Protestant reform, the Puritan struggle encompassed a number of issues—parliamentary rule and royal prerogative, religious observance and celebration, and most important, hair. The Puritans believed that England's commitment to the Reformation did not go deep enough: Papal influences still held sway in the Church hierarchy, paganism among the peasants. Only local teachers could bring the word of

God close enough to the ears of individual sinners, and only strict adherence to the codes of godly behavior would make it intelligible. Royalists and peasants alike were given to distracting amusements—May Day celebrations that included mixed dancing, bowling, drinking, and hunting. The Puritan man took commitment to the godly life seriously and literally: he believed in the sanctity of the Sabbath, the holiness of sober industry, and the righteousness of short hair.

Though there were certainly notable exceptions—Oliver Cromwell, for example, wore his hair long—the association of Puritans with short hair was prevalent in the middle of the seventeenth century in England, and even spawned a somewhat derogatory nickname: Roundhead. The Puritan press dubbed Cavaliers agents of "popery and profanation" given to licentiousness and vice. Themselves given to wearing "Prince Rupert's locks," long and curly, Cavaliers scorned the Roundheads for their haircuts and boring insistence on sobriety. One poet maintained that the Roundheads had ruined Christmas, since they believed that "roast beef was anti-Christian and that mince pies were the relics of the Whore of Babylon." Dr. Martin Mar-Prelat wrote a sympathetic verse in 1640 describing a Puritan, "As They Are Now Termed by Profane Atheists, etc.": "A Puritan is he . . . Whose Hair, and Ruffs, dare not his Ears exceed: that on high Saints' days wears his Working Weed." Disciplined, industrious, literate, and persecuted by the crown: the Puritans were the perfect settlers for a new world colony where their own ethics—of dress, work, and religion—would set the standards and English investors would reap the benefits.

In the earliest days of American settlement, Parliamentary struggle was almost irrelevant, but religion was not. Faced with the opportunity to establish what future Massachusetts Bay governor John Winthrop imagined as a "Modell of Christian Charitie" on the coast of New England, America's Puritan settlers were perhaps even more zealously committed to reform than they had been before. In the scattered towns of earliest settlement—Salem, Watertown, Charlestown, Boston—church membership was only for the elect, those who had shown proper and visible signs of being saved by the Lord, and participation in the government of the town depended on church membership. Community life, then, was bound on all sides by the religious aspirations of the Puritan movement.

In my second grade Thanksgiving play, we stood behind a brown boat cut from cardboard and recounted the story of the pilgrims: their fearful flight from a torturous England, the difficulties of piety in a passive Holland, their celebration of religious freedom in the New World we were fortunate enough to inhabit as their progeny. The truth is, though, that these pilgrims were not at all interested in religious freedom as we imagine it today; what they wanted was complete and total control.

John Calvin's doctrine of predestination provided the New England colonies with a basis for their lofty ideals and for their own special brand of spiritual paranoia. Despite His grave disappointment with human behavior, God had chosen certain people to reside with Him in Heaven; the rest were condemned to Hell. Since God was omnipotent, there was no possibility for human alteration of His choice. Indeed, human life was almost irrelevant to the entire business of election and damnation, except that it might serve as a setting for the demonstration of God's will. The elect would certainly lead righteous and holy lives and serve as examples to others of the power and goodness of God. But since the damned might also choose to imitate the goodness of the elect, the true drama of life would be the assessment of earthly claims to heavenly election, the separation of the *seemingly* good from the *truly* good. New England's Puritans certainly intended to construct a community of the elect, and they certainly believed that election was not something human intervention could alter—it was a free choice of God's, made before an individual could affect any influence—but they could not bring themselves to give up on social regulation and civil rule, which might indeed be superfluous in a true gathering of saved individuals, but which their years in England had taught them were necessary for a holy life on Earth.

So, woven into the very fabric of New England's foundation, there was a series of grave, unsolvable conflicts: Why is it necessary to regulate what is supposed to be voluntary, free, and entirely in the hands of God? How is it possible to assess that which can solely be determined by the will of God at the end of days? If Puritan life seems a mass of contradictions and self-flagellations, it was because they had bound themselves to live by a philosophy that purported to offer the ultimate guidance but in reality offered very little. Endless scrutiny, then, became the Puritan answer to their spiritual bind—regulation, determination, and minute examination, of oneself and of one's peers. Membership in the church required not only that an individual be saved, but that they prove their salvation—as far as anyone could prove an unknowable premise—to the elders of the church through word, deed, and deportment. When the ships carrying the Massachusetts Bay settlers missed Virginia and drifted north to Plymouth instead, the Bay Company leaders were relieved; they'd heard the Virginians were a godless bunch and had feared life among them. But when they tried to join the worship at the Plymouth church, they encountered for the first time the stringencies of the New World's Puritans. Unable to "prove" their election, they were left to worship on their own.

Sumptuary laws, laws governing the use of luxury items, became a mainstay of colonial morality—ambivalently worded codes begging for an order that should have been easier to maintain. Designed to curb the taste for luxury that was undermining the humble philosophy of the colonies and, at the same time, straining the delicate balance of social hierarchy, sumptuary laws were passed in the earliest years of the colonies and were enforced through most of the seventeenth century. In September, 1634, the Massachusetts General Court outlawed "greate, superfluous & unnecessary expences occacioned by reason of some new & immodest fashions." Men and women of "meane condition" were not to wear "gold or silver lace, or buttons, or poynts at theire kneese," and poorer women were forbidden to don "silke or tiffany hoodes or scarfes." The magistrates spoke out in 1649 against other fashions they believed were luring New Englanders to the devil's court. Long hair was one of their primary concerns. "[T]he wearing of long haire after the manner of Ruffians and barbarous Indians hath begun to invade New England contrary to the rule of God's word," they warned. It is "uncivil and unmanly wherby men doe deform themselves, and offend sober & modest men, & does corrupt good manners."

Women and Harvard College students were of special concern in the controversy over hair fashions. One minister lamented, "The special sin of women is pride and haughtiness, and that because they are generally ignorant and worthless." Another worried that their hairstyles clouded his ministerial judgement. "And lest it should fall down, it is under propped with forks, wiers, and I cannot tell what, like grim sterne monsters, rather than chaste Christian matrones." Like flighty women, Harvard students seemed given to fashion fancies that were unbecoming of humble students of the Lord. Before the college was two decades old, President Charles Chauncy announced a strict dress code that included a list of prohibited hair fashions. Students were forbidden "Long Haire, Locks or foretopps, nor to use Curling, Crispings, parting or powdering their haire."

Michael Wigglesworth, minister of Malden, gave an admonitory sermon to the unrepentant students that might have been given three centuries later to Berkeley hippies. "That length of hair which is womanish and savors of effeminacy is unlawfull," he argued. "*You are bound to imitate the generality of the best. Why wil you do it in this country, where most of the people of God wear short hair?*" Finally, he urges them to conform for their own sake. "Walk safely," he begs. "If there be a sin in long hair certain it is no sin to wear short hair; chuse that which is most safe."

Ezekiel Rogers of Rowley cut short his nephew's inheritance because the young man refused to live with his uncle, dropped out of Harvard, and "because he spoke to his mother to have his haire cutt but could not get it done." Oddly enough, his mother supported his decision not to cut his long hair as well as his decision to contest his uncle's will. She told her minister she would "never yield to such a snare for her child, tho' he never had a penny of his while he lived."

If Papists and Cavaliers hovered in the background of Puritan hair controversies, Indians loomed large in the foreground, both as a physical threat to the colonists' security and as a bad but riveting example of moral laxity. New England leaders blamed the colonists' "backslidings from God" for King Philip's War in 1675, the bloodiest conflict of the colonial era, and in a frenzy of spiritual reckoning outlined their grievances in tightened fashion regulations. "Vaine, new, strange fashions . . . with naked breasts and armes" and "superstitious ribbons both on haire and apparrell" were signs that the colonists had abandoned God. Another was that "long haire, like weomens haire, is worne by some men, either their oune or others haire made into perewiggs, and by some women wearing borders of haire, and theire cutting curling, & imodest laying out of theire haire . . ." The deadliness of the war and a continued feeling of insecurity was a sign that God had likewise abandoned the colonists. A generation later, Nicholas Noyes, a Salem minister who wrote a long and scathing essay against the wearing of periwigs, thought concern with hair fashions a dangerous irony in a place where Indians lurked on the borders anxious to remove the colonists' scalps. "Alas," he cried, "that men should be so prodigal and profuse this way in an age so barren . . . and when they are so much needed for the maintaining [of] the government . . . and for building forts, and maintaining soldiers to defend the plantation against enemies that will take off the scalp, both skin and hair . . ."

Like the witches who had taken up residence within the colonies themselves, Indians seemed a spiritual test of New England's fitness for God's favor. A profligate bunch, who lived without benefit of sacrament, industry, or learning, the Indians seemed impervious to their own spiritual peril. They steadfastly refused to improve their land, preferring instead to live without fences and migrate with the seasons; their women farmed while the men amused themselves with rich men's sport—hunting, fishing, and sex. Their fashion sense was particularly barbarous, since in most seasons they were almost naked, and their hair—long, greased, and decorated—belied an utterly unwarranted pride. John Eliot, whom Cotton Mather dubbed the "Apostle to the Indians," praised those who had adopted Christianity with the help of Puritan ministers, and "have discerned the vanitie and pride which they placed in their haire and have therefore of their own accord . . . cut it modestly." The Christian Indians of Nonantum established a tax of five shillings on long hair for men and short hair for women. For Indians and Puritans alike, adherence to Paul's hair rules was a sign of submission, to the "yoke of Christ," and also to the Puritans.

In the colonists' absence, England had adopted the French men's fashion for wigs—long, elaborate, and usually greased with oil, lard, or bear grease and powdered with flour. Gradually, the wigs spread to the colonies, where they were widely worn and just as widely excoriated. Along with many of his peers, Nicholas Noyes worried that wigs tampered with the perfection of God's work, upsetting the gender balance so explicitly elaborated by Paul, since men's wigs were often manufactured from women's hair cut from the heads of live women. "It seems to be unlawful and most foolish and absurd for a woman to part with her hair to adorn a man," wrote Noyes. "If the hair of women be so necessary and useful as it is pretended in this age, for periwigs, perhaps the next age may find a way to spin it and make cloth of it. And their skins, well tanned, may make good leather; and at length they will become very profitable creatures to men." Like the rebellious youth of the 1960s, Noyes considered wigs despicable disguises. "A man with his hair cut off, and another's put on, looketh not as he did before . . ." he reasoned. Most important, as a disguise and as a pretension to youth, the periwig exacerbated the difficulties already plaguing the Calvinist project. Fashionable masks might further obscure spiritual deficiencies and render the entire society unintelligible. "When gray hairs are removed out of sight," warned Noyes, ". . . it hath a natural tendency to make men forget that they stand upon the edge of the grave and on the brink of Eternity."

Though his son Cotton wore one, Increase Mather, formidable pastor of Boston's Great North Church, deplored wigs as "Horrid Bushes of Vanity." Cotton, for his part, dismissed the entire debate. Those who wasted time railing against wigs, he thought, "strained at a gnat and swallowed a camel."

As the eighteenth century wore on, wigs progressed from

a spiritual problem to a symbol of the increasingly burden-some political, social, and economic ties to England. The same was true of women's hairstyles, which were con-structed from false hair stretched over padded wire "rolls," and were often elaborate headdresses adorned with flowers, jewels, and tiny toys. Often, these constructions were held in place with grease, like men's wigs and the bouffants of the 1950s, and then powdered; they could last for weeks, as long as the lady in question slept sitting up and took care not to knock into doorways, low-hanging branches, or other dangers. Numerous cartoons of the period depict the absurdity of eighteenth-century ladies' hair fashions: hair-dressers perched on ladders, deploying toy boats in a three-foot sea of hair; carriages with lowered floors or open roofs, specifically designed to accommodate madame's towering coif.

To the republican leaders of America, the sartorial extravagance of fanciful wigs and elaborate coiffures sig-naled the decadence of a colonial society slavishly devoted to imitating the corrupt habits of the motherland. Austerity measures meant to recover lost republican virtue were also inherently rebellious rejections of British goods, attention, and control. Women were urged to forego imported silk and to wear dresses made from homespun; boycotts of tea and other "taxables" galvanized a spirit of collective market virtue. Though wigs and high headdressings did not disap-pear immediately, and indeed they remained the subject of great debate and public scorn, their folly was sometimes turned to political purpose. Republican barbers were known to sabotage the wigs of their Tory clients, and in the midst of the conflict, some women wore their hair in a series of thirteen rolls, a tribute to the thirteen colonies dubbed *à l'independence* in proper French fashion. When the rebel forces retook Philadelphia in 1778, a rowdy street parade showed their disapproval of the lingering pre–Revolutionary War hairstyles by displaying a "very dirty woman" wearing a "very high Head dress," who was followed through the streets "with a mob after her, with drums &c by way of ridiculing that very foolish fashion."

John Adams hoped that the revolution would "have this good Effect, at least: it will inspire Us with many Virtues, which We have not, and correct many Errors, Follies and Vices." And indeed, in the aftermath of the revolution, hair fashions simplified considerably, though slowly. Some of the founding fathers wore wigs, but did without powder; some wore powder, but would not wear wigs. By the 1820s, men's wigs had disappeared—hairpieces became "invisible" after this—and women's hair was styled low and close to the head, parted around the face to highlight the sincerity of a gentle countenance. And yet, the struggle over republican fashion virtue has lingered throughout America's history: it is the spiritual crisis of the Puritans translated into the language of the Enlightenment. In pursuit of social virtue, republicans in all ages have advocated sartorial modesty and tonsorial honesty—a strict correlation between outward appearance and inner reality. Luxury hints at disguise, and disguise at vice. And vice hints, always, at damnation.

Men do not demand genuine beauty, even in the most modest doses; they are quite content with the mere appearance of beauty. That is to say, they show no talent whatever for differentiating between the artificial and the real. . . . The hair of a dead Chinaman, artfully dressed and dyed, gives them as much delight as the authentic tresses of Venus.

—H. L. Mencken, "In Defense of Women"

The hair revolution of the 1920s may have been a reprisal of the 1660s, or a foreshadowing of what was to come in the 1960s. It was certainly stunning and acrimonious enough, except for one crucial detail: now, instead of men seeming to shirk the responsibilities of masculine restraint by wearing their hair long, it seemed women were attempting to usurp them by wearing their hair short. During one frenzied week of 1924, 3,500 women had their hair bobbed in one New York salon, where the stylists kept smelling salts close at hand because so many women fainted when they saw their hair fall away from their heads. "I must say that first snip of the scissors gave me a shock," remembered one woman, "like a cold bath or taking gas." Despite frequent rumors of its demise, however, the bob only became more popular as the decade wore on and the initial shock wore off. By 1925, fifty-three percent of Mount Holyoke's students had bobbed their hair. Soon, rumors began to spread in New York: it was said that in Paris, "they're showing their ears."

Perhaps the bob was the perfect statement for an ambivalent, manic decade when so much of America seemed to change so fast. In 1920, one out of thirteen Americans owned a car—traffic lights were invented just in time. Prohibition, suffrage for women, the Scopes Trial and Lindenberg's transatlantic flight followed the end of World War I in rapid succession, turning what Americans imagined had

27

been a static, safe world into a whirling centrifuge. To many, it seemed a shaky era of false appearances. The Volstead Act had made it illegal to manufacture, transport, or sell alcohol, but not to purchase or consume it, so America's alcohol simply disappeared from plain view. Hidden behind heavily paneled doors drilled with peepholes, it seemed to flow freely from springs concealed just beneath the surface of American life. It took one Prohibition agent only thirty-five seconds to find a drink in New Orleans.

A vibrant youth culture emerged in the thick of the conflict, taking advantage of the freedom and mobility of modern life. Like their 1960s counterparts, the youth of the 1920s worked together to shed the fetters of their parents' generation, calling on the newly translated Freud to push for what author Ben Lindsey deemed "sexual honesty." *Harper's* reported that this generation "exalts sincerity, truth, naturalness." Fashion was an integral part of this search for authenticity and freedom: shorter skirts and sleeves meant female limbs could move without hindrance; exposed flesh and visible makeup boldly claimed sexual purpose. Corsets, petticoats, and garters, all binding restraints, were tossed aside, and, with the aid of a succession of fad diets, a new physique emerged. Long, slim, and sleek, the flapper's body could run, shake, and shimmy without shame.

The flapper's hair fit easily into this energetic ideal. Cropped and close, it had been liberated from the knots, stays, and falsely padded pompadours of previous years, and emitted the sexual charge usually associated with "loose" hair. At the same time, it evoked an androgynous charm that might have muted its threat in another age. The variety of names given bobbed styles—the Garçon, the Coconut, and Gigolo—emphasized that playful, boyish edge, and magazines like *Good Housekeeping* celebrated it for its simplicity and ease, but reaction was swift and blustery nonetheless.

Charles Nessler, hair guru and inventor of the permanent wave machine, warned that if women kept cutting their hair they would weaken the scalp muscles and eventually begin to bald like men. The superintendent of schools in Constantine, Michigan, dismissed the entire flapper ethos. "I can see no place in society for bobbed hair, dresses that do not cover the knee, and like contraptions," he snapped. When a judge asked the oldest child of one Missouri woman whose children had been placed in foster care if she'd like to return to her mother, the twelve-year-old girl declined adamantly. "We don't believe Mother is a Christian woman," she said. "And the Bible says in the eleventh chapter of First Corinthians that a woman should not cut her hair." And, she added, "She wears jewelry and bright clothes." A tract that asked, "Bobbed Hair: Is it well-pleasing to the Lord?" noted that short hair was part of a larger trend of feminine rebellion. Women everywhere were suddenly refusing to say "obey" in the marriage ceremony, and were seen smoking in public. For its British readers familiar with Paul's letter, the pamphlet did some much-needed translating, noting that " 'bobbed' is only another way of saying shorn . . ." One Pennsylvania school board awarded a hundred-dollar bonus to teachers who left their hair long.

Some colleges passed sumptuary rules against bobbed hair, makeup, and cigarettes, but student pressure and the wild popularity of the trend made such efforts weak at best. In 1925, an Ohio State student paper estimated that seventy percent of the university's female students had bobbed hair. The rest, it remarked, "belong to the old brigade." Screen star Lynn Fontanne recommended bobbed hair and makeup to all *Ladies Home Journal* readers. "Long hair is dangerously on the edge of frumpishness," she observed. Even little Mary Pickford, who hemmed and hawed for months, eventually cropped her girlish waves, admitting that "smartness" was currently more important than "beauty." And when rumors predicted the return of long hair, members of the newly expanded hairdressing profession fought back with scarcely veiled threats. Joseph de Silvis, who claimed to have invented the bob, warned, "If we take a good look at those who are starting to let their hair grow, we feel sorry for them. . . . They are fidgety and develop a terrible nervous condition."

Thirteen years after the repeal of Prohibition and the stock market crash had effectively ended the twenties and its compulsive gaiety, Ernest Hemingway began work on *The Garden of Eden*, a novel that must have drawn and troubled him, since he worked on it for fifteen more years, until his death, without finishing it. The story of expatriate Americans who wander from France to Spain and back again in unhurried haste, *The Garden of Eden* is in many ways a typical Hemingway tale of alienation and alcoholism. Except that *The Garden of Eden* benefits more than most Hemingway novels from the acuity of hindsight—it has the aura of a parable, as if it was meant to be a morality tale for an era only remembered by a passing generation. That's why it is so significant that Hemingway's story gathers its momentum from a series of haircuts. When Catherine Bourne, the stunning new wife of writer David Bourne, decides to crop her hair—shorter than a bob, even—we begin to have an inkling of trouble to come. She's gone further than the frivolous flappers of New York, and her recklessness bodes immediately of danger, of boundaries not just crossed but violated. "It was cut with no compromises," she tells David. "That's the surprise. I'm a girl. But now I'm a boy too and I can do anything and anything and anything."

Over time, Catherine's hair gets shorter and lighter, her skin darker and darker. She pushes David to have his hair cut just like hers, then lightened to match. When they take another woman into their marriage, it is clear that the Bournes' union is like their hair—cropped beyond recognition and stripped of color. Their roles—masculine, feminine, helpmeet—have lost their roots, and at the same time, their meaning. After Catherine Bourne's first visit to the hairdresser, the French villagers gather for a peek at her exotic coif. Firmly ensconced in the domestic safety of the forties and fifties, Hemingway has remembered the essence of the twenties in a single, devastating act—the cutting of a woman's hair. He wrote, "No decent girls had ever had their hair cut short like that in this part of the country and even in Paris it was rare and strange and could be beautiful or could be very bad."

A Final Word: Hair Revolutions on the Eve of the Millennium

The crisis of the late sixties and early seventies faded as the end of Nixon's presidency erased the great divide between youth activists and grown-up pragmatists. Suddenly, political cynicism was a necessity and hair wars were plainly irrelevant. When the young men of Generation X grew their hair into long slick ponytails, few could be bothered to disturb the calm pool of the Reagan era and protest. What good would it have done? The suspicion of the seventies combined with the placid self-interest of the eighties to foster an apathy to the politics of fashion. The sixties and seventies haunt our fashion runways, but the spirit of protest has seemingly fled. As we face the millennium our fashion gurus are in a frenzy of historic curiosity, but each adaptation is merely that—a two-dimensional cutout with a hole for our faces to smile through for the camera. In the 1990s we focus on style—Jennifer Aniston's shag, the revival of Audrey Hepburn's pixie, the hundred-dollar blowout that turns curly hair bone straight.

Quietly, though, our own hair revolution has been brewing. The brazen spirit of the Afro, which claimed to celebrate the unique texture of black hair and black heritage, has been resurrected in the braids and locks of the 1990s. And though there has been no groundswell of protest against these now ubiquitous styles, a certain amount of corporate *stalling* has landed a number of cases in court, where Title VII protections have had to compete with the inflated exigencies of company dress codes. The original spate of lawsuits, brought in the late eighties and early nineties, involved airlines and hotels, organizations that imagined customer comfort could not include a customer service agent with braids. More recently, the scope of offending corporations has expanded to include a parking company and the Washington, D.C., police force, where an officer with locks was threatened with removal from the force if he did not change his hairstyle.

Diane Seltzer, the Washington lawyer for Jeff Robinson, the D.C. police officer, doesn't talk about karma and kismet and other universal forces that make the right things happen, but she finds some meaning in her client's arriving in her office when he did. A nice Jewish girl from New York, Seltzer is no stranger to hair trauma. She remembers being relieved at summer camp because everyone else there was Jewish, and her curly hair wasn't the anomaly it was at her school in the city. "I wanted to be like the non-Jewish girls and have straight hair," she says now, admitting that some of her sympathy for Jeff Robinson might have roots in her childhood. But her real devotion to the case comes from the murder of a good friend of hers on the weekend of Yom Kippur in 1996. The D.C. police followed few, if any of the proper procedures for handling his case—"They botched it," says Seltzer—and now, three years later, they have not come close to solving the crime. In the meantime, this earnest, accomplished young officer was being punished for growing his hair in locks in accordance with his religious beliefs (he has taken the vow of the Nazarites and will not cut his hair, drink wine, or handle a dead body). To Selzter, the contrast between the shoddy investigation and the overzealous attention to a good cop's personal grooming seemed to epitomize everything that was wrong with the department.

Even to legal neophytes like myself, Robinson's case seems easily decided. Religion and personal appearance are both protected by civil rights laws in Washington, and Robinson easily explains how his locks make him a more accessible presence on the streets. At least nine other officers on the force, including Robinson's current captain, wear their hair in locks. Only one of them has had any problems, and his seem, legally anyway, to have come to an end. Seltzer herself is shocked that the case has gone this far—the trial is approaching, and despite an injunction forbidding the force from disciplining Robinson, the police department seems unconcerned about the weakness of its case. "He just wanted to do his job," says Seltzer. "There's so much crime in this city, and this is what they're doing?" Seltzer can't do anything to help her friend, and she can't do much to solve his murder, but she's determined to make Robinson's case part of her healing. "The only thing I can do is help a policeman who wants to be a policeman." Whatever the resolution of the case, Robinson isn't sure that he can envision a future for himself on the force; he doesn't think that he'll be made a detective after all of this is over—he's caused too much trouble for the department. He's been talking to friends about other businesses he might get into—maybe real estate, or car stereos or alarms.

If Diane Seltzer is the "Queen of Locks" in D.C. legal circles, Eric Steele is proud to call himself the king. His relationship to this hair crisis is long and involved, going back a decade already; he's handled braids cases against American Airlines, the Washington Hyatt, Marriott, and the Boston Harbor Hotel, and he has two locks cases pending, one against Household Finance and another against a Tennessee-based company that owns public garages, Central Parking. Disney phoned him once, asking for advice on getting rid of their policy against employees wearing braids. Steele laughs as he admits that he wasn't as flip as he wanted to be. "I wanted to tell them to take their red pens, cross it out, send it to the printer, and redistribute." A number of the companies he's fought have had similar policies, a fact that frustrates and amuses Steele, but has not kept his cases out of court. "Some pinhead from all these companies put it in there. The truth is, most people don't read their handbook." And it is not legal to forbid an aesthetic that is associated primarily with one racial or ethnic group. Indeed, it was in a protective response to the Afro that this interpretation of Title VII evolved. "You don't have the right to wear [your hair] to your ankles," says Steele, "but the employer doesn't have the right to ban braids entirely either."

Over the course of his lengthy experience with employment litigation and hair discrimination, Steele has developed a vocabulary that belies a certain humorous weariness—there is no excuse or plan for settlement he has not heard before. American Airlines tried to convince the court that while *natural* hairstyles, like the Afro, might be protected under Title VII, braids are not *natural*, they are a choice, and therefore not protected. "You have to be from Mars for that to make sense," he says, laughing. In another case, they conceded that braids would be allowed on the job, but that the employee would have to cover them with a scarf or something like it. Steele calls that the "Aunt Jemima Revision." When one of their lawyers argued that the no-braids policy was inspired by the movie *10*, in which a white Bo Derek wears her hair in long cornrows, and was not in any way meant to discriminate against African Americans, Steele was skeptical and said so. Now, he thunders at the memory. "What if I said *you* all had to wear *Afros!*" Just the thought makes him laugh again.

Still, despite the fact that by his own estimate he and

Diane Selzter handle most of the personal appearance discrimination cases in Washington, Steele doesn't see himself as a crusader. He wouldn't want to handle any upcoming safety-pin-in-the-nose cases, he says. Hair discrimination makes much better legal sense.

Three

∫Uncommon Pains
Tales of African Hair in America

It is three days before Valentine's Day, and I am expecting Marcelle's braiding salon in the Fort Greene section of Brooklyn to be packed. But it is nearly empty; Marcelle has been closed for three months because of an accident involving her baby daughter, and this is her first day back on the job. Shyly, she waves to the people who knock on the window and greet her, people who are glad to see that another neighborhood business has not closed for good and that Marcelle has not decided to leave Fort Greene.

Nancy, a fortysomething grandmother who is Marcelle's only client for the day, is having a new weave put in. Standing straight behind Nancy's seat, Marcelle is not much taller than her sitting customer, and through the plate glass window at the front of the salon, she appears slightly magical, as if she is performing secret rituals on Nancy's tilted head. With a curved blunt needle and sturdy black thread she attaches wefts—hair sewn into a line to form a sort of panel—to Nancy's own hair, which is braided in cornrows close to her head. This process will allow Nancy to cover her own hair without having to bear the close cap of a wig. The hair in the wefts is long and the wefts are sewn close together, so after four or five are attached, it looks as if Nancy has shoulder length "bone straight" hair—black with red-gold highlights, because every other weft is blond and Nancy is not one to settle for monochrome.

To Nancy, her own hair is not as interesting as the hair she wears in her weave. In fact, she's been wearing a weave for ten years straight now, and she's not even entirely sure she knows her own hair. She speaks about it as she would a sickly plant or a wayward adolescent in need of rehabilitation. Marcelle is careful with Nancy's hair so that it remains healthy underneath the weave. "My hair grows for her," Nancy says, not sure she has the touch herself. She'd like to maybe wear it in a perm, but she's not sure what would happen. "If I try to perm it now, it'll go *aak*!" She cries out in rebellion, perhaps even pain. "My hair's been in lockdown for ten years . . ." It's not ready for the outside world.

Next summer, she vows with the solemnity of a choco-holic who feels fat on New Year's Eve, she'll start wearing her own hair. She'll take out her weave, let her hair "relax" for a while, then perm the front and get a weave in back. This way, she can wear her own hair without giving up the length and versatility she gets with the weave. "I like my hair wild," she says, smiling to herself. "With my own hair, I can't be wild."

Marcelle, whose business consists mainly of the latest trends—weaves, braids, twists—thinks she understands these new styles. In part, she concedes, what makes a weave essential to someone like Nancy is dissatisfaction, a discomfort with what is already there. Black Europeans go to the beauty shop much less often than African Americans, because they are much less concerned with their hair. Marcelle, who was born in Senegal, reared in Marseilles, and has worked in Paris, Frankfurt, and Africa, thinks that African Americans have "suffered a lot. They've been mocked. They were taught that their hair was ugly, it was nappy. . . . So they feel the need to go to the beauty shop more often. What's most important to them is the hair." For Europeans, she says, it's the clothes.

And yet, like almost everyone involved in the business of braiding, twisting, and weaving, Marcelle is quick to point out the natural, organic relationship between black people and the latest black styles. Braids, twists, and weaves are part of an African heritage, a set of practices that stretch back across oceans and more than four thousand years. Even though many typically African styles are "too much" (i.e., too elaborate) for her American customers, Marcelle sees her work as part of a continuum, a strategy for long-term cultural survival. It is also a practical endeavor. Styles such as Silky Dreds, where individual braids are wrapped tight with shiny synthetic hair, may be a little painful at first—one woman described it as having a "head full of pencils"—but they can last for several months, saving time, money, and energy for the customer. Though braided styles can cost anywhere from $75 to $600, most agree that they are better values, in the long run, than perms and relaxers. Far kinder to the hair than straightening chemicals and hot combs, which can burn the scalp and cause hair loss, they are also easier to maintain, eliminating lengthy morning maintenance rituals. "We're looking for what is practical, what is easier," says Marcelle. "All of us."

It's very American, this emphasis on practicality, convenience, ease on the way to the office. But for Marcelle, *American* is an ambivalent term, full of promise and limitation. Arriving in New York City nine years ago at age twenty-six, Marcelle expected paradise. She imagined New York as the society of the future: a racially integrated boomtown, with fifteen-lane highways and luxurious skyscrapers that even the most sybaritic tenant would never have to leave. What she found was a not-so-integrated city where skyscrapers are bank offices, not luxury dwellings, and the face of poverty is decidedly dark. "When I came here, the first thing I learned was that people look at you first through your color. I was shocked: I thought I had more to offer than that."

Marcelle is relieved to have African restaurants so close to her home, because many days she comes home too exhausted to cook for her three children, but she admits to being surprised that a combination of economics and demographics steered her so steadily toward a black neighborhood. "If you're black, here, then you'll be in a black neighborhood," she says, frustration edging her quiet voice. "I was disappointed because I never had to live that way." Her thoughts echo the wails of turn-of-the-century immigrants blindsided by the realization that the streets of New York were not paved in gold after all. She wasn't prepared for a racially divided life, and she wasn't prepared for New York's unforgiving economy. "We were given the United States of Dr. Martin Luther

King," she says, turning her story into an African morality tale. "We thought all Americans had milk delivered every morning."

Bound on one side by East River shipyards, and by Atlantic, Flatbush, and Vanderbilt Avenues on the others, Fort Greene is a neighborhood of Old New York—both orderly and chaotic, proud and decrepit. The first European to make Fort Greene his home, Peter Caesar Alberti, planted tobacco. His successors built ships. Drawn by the prospect of skilled work, free blacks began to arrive in the area in the 1840s, at the same time that Frederick Law Olmsted, famed author of Central Park, created Washington Park (later called Fort Greene Park), the rolling centerpiece of the neighborhood. By the 1870s, more than half the black population of Brooklyn had settled in Fort Greene.

The streets that surround Marcelle's shop are lined with rows of Queen Anne brownstones, more delicate and lean than their Upper West Side counterparts and far more exquisite. But residents often shake their heads when asked about the evolution of their neighborhood. It was safe once, they say, safe enough to send your son to the corner store by himself with a dollar for some milk. No one does that now. Though the avenues are lined with businesses—African shops, Hispanic restaurants, cleverly named hardware stores—and Fort Greene has by no means succumbed to the poverty that has made neighborhoods like Bedford-Stuyvesant notorious, the occasional abandoned storefront makes clear what residents rarely forget: however picturesque, Fort Greene is largely a black neighborhood and its fortunes depend on the earning power of a disadvantaged population. Even on a gray February day, Fort Greene seems like a nice place to live, but it is not prime real estate.

Despite her discouragement, Marcelle plans to see what New York will offer in the twenty-first century. She and her fellow West Africans, many of whom have settled around her in Fort Greene, and many of whom try to make a living braiding hair, are still in love with the possibilities of America. "We all have better lives in Africa," she admits. "But it's the dream. Something better *has* to happen."

"Lately Imported from Africa"

For the owners of the four hundred thousand Africans forcibly brought to North America between 1619 and 1808, when the transatlantic traffic in humans was supposed to have ended, a slave's hair was a small but crucial piece of property. Indeed, it grew from the uppermost portion of what happened to be a substantial investment. Depending on their health, their age, their sex, their temperament, and their skills, a slave could cost anywhere from a few hundred to a few thousand dollars in early America; a slave's hair—like her teeth or her feet—served as an indicator of suitability, a sign of what tasks the slave's body could be expected to perform. For this reason, prospective sellers plucked gray hairs from the heads of slaves they were hoping to sell, and Robert Roberts's *House Servant's Directory* (1827) advised every home to have a "safe liquid" for the purpose of dying slave hair the deep black it was supposed to be. William Wells Brown, a former slave, called this "the blacking process," and claimed that it could make a slave appear fifteen years younger than he was.

Few slaves could read, and even fewer could write, or had the means and motivation to record their feelings, so we have only scant, refracted information about how slaves themselves approached their hair. The South Carolina Negro Act of 1735 designated certain rough cloths with broguish names—kearsies, osnabrigs, and linsey-woolsies—the only legal material for slave clothing. Wary of the effect of gentlemen's garments on a slave's habit of servitude, the South Carolina legislature also restricted the style of clothing a slave was allowed to wear. In theory, at least, slaves were no longer permitted to wear castoffs from their owners' closets, and authorities would confiscate any clothing thought to befit persons of a higher rank. And yet, the very existence of such a law indicates the difficulty of policing the attire of slaves. In ads pleading for the return of runaways, slave owners often described the clothing the slave was known to have taken. Many times, the escaped slaves possessed items of prohibited finery, such as cast-off coats, shoes, and bonnets, possibly provided as part of a house slave's livery, or given as a reward for sexual favors. A slave named Jenny, who ran from her Philadelphia master in 1782, took with her "blue worsted shoes with white heels," as well as "a new black peelong bonnet." Jenny must have been a favorite of his, because he also noted that she was "particularly fond" of "queen's night caps."

As part of their general appearance, a slave's hair was also something to be controlled and regulated. Although laws did not specify particular styles allowed to the slave, in the eighteenth century and well into the nineteenth century, wigs were the attire of gentlemen, and were thus a controversial, if not prohibited, part of a slave's wardrobe. House slaves had at their disposal better grooming supplies and conditions than their fieldworking peers, but they also lived more closely under the watchful eyes of their masters. Their hair might be better kept—others noted that it was often "combed" and sometimes "greased with lard" or tucked under a clean white kerchief—but it was also at higher risk. Some plantation mistresses, jealous of the attention their husbands gave certain female slaves, punished both the slaves and their husbands by having the slave's long, presumably alluring, hair cut off. Male slaves, less likely to use their hair to overstep their place on the plantation, were more likely to be dressed as women and paraded as sissies for punishment, or to have their heads dunked in buckets of lye. (According to some sources, the side effects of this punishment prompted the development of lye-based commercial straightening formulas.)

Like many slave traditions, the braiding, shaving, and wrapping techniques of American slaves originated in Africa, where they were important rituals of distinction. European travelers in Africa described the "fantastic coiffures" of the natives: plaits decorated with shells, beads, cloth; heads shaved in the front, on the sides, or in the back. Egyptian wigs made from grass, fiber, and human hair sit in cases in our museums, where the climate is carefully controlled so that they do not deteriorate. In 1456, Cado Mosto described African men and women with hair woven into "beautiful tresses, which they tie in various knots, though it be very short." Recounting his travels in Guinea, Pieter de Marees, a Dutch explorer, published an illustration of sixteen hairstyles from Benin. Some depict hair shaped into multipronged crowns, while others seem almost Roman, short styles with bangs topped with laurel leaves. In West Africa, Yoruba shaving rituals marked both the beginning and the end of life, and young boys had their heads shaved on the sides.

It may be easy for the modern reader to see the signs of continuity, since the braids of one country can easily resemble the plaits of another. But it is easy, too, to see the mark of pragmatism on the heads of slaves. The ubiquitous kerchief, a staple of the field hand's wardrobe and a hallmark of Hollywood mammies, might have recalled the customs of the Gold Coast Ashanti, who are supposed to have had over fifty names for kerchief styles, but it also must have kept the dust out of hair that was not easily cared for in the life of a southern slave who had neither time nor energy nor grooming supplies. And yet, runaway slave ads and other accounts belie the notion that grooming itself was a haphazard, random act for the enslaved individual.

One eighteenth-century observer watched recent captives gather on the deck of a ship in Suriname, moons and stars shaved into their heads. They had used soap and pieces of broken glass to decorate each other, since they were not provided with razors during the Middle Passage to the West. We know that along with kerchiefs and wrapping rags and strings—bits of cloth and string used like modern curlers—slaves made combs for themselves out of cow horns and corncobs. Sundays, the only "free" day for plantation slaves, were often used for grooming and display. It was the day the kerchief came off and the slave barber's razor came out. An ad for a slave named Bazil, who ran away from a Maryland plantation in the 1780s, remarks on his "woolly hair, in which he takes great pride." The owner of a "Negro Man called Dick," who fled from his New Jersey home in June of 1770, claimed that Dick was "about five feet eight inches high, about 28 years of age," spoke "very good English," and was a "well-looking, well-built fellow, somewhat on the Yellow." Dick was also known to take "uncommon Pains with his short woolly Hair, which he wears cut on the fore Part of his Head."

Frances Kemble, a British actress who was dismayed to discover that her new husband's Georgia plantation was worked by over seven hundred slaves, hoped that the slaves' attention to appearance might bode well for the possibility of acculturation. "The passion for dress is curiously strong in these people," she wrote in 1863, "and seems as though it might be made an instrument in converting them." Signs of adopted white mores were encouraging, even if in contrast they highlighted what Kemble perceived to be the monstrosity of black fashion. "Though their own native taste is decidedly both barbarous and ludicrous," she writes, "it is astonishing how very soon they mitigate it in imitation of white models." Indeed, just as it is relatively easy to trace the influence of African hairdressing on the practices of Southern slaves, it is almost equally easy to point to what might be termed "white influences," or the incorporation of European standards and techniques. Stolen wigs and coiffures like that of the New York runaway Prince, who wore his hair "tied up behind, and a large tupee before," hint that the gentleman's peruke might have had a special appeal for the oppressed male slave. Photographs of free black or runaway abolitionists from the middle years of the nineteenth century show women with tightly drawn buns and careful chignons, men with close-cropped waves, mustaches, and side parts. Frederick Douglass, abolitionist, memoirist, and publisher, his gray hair a highstanding mane, was the exception, not the rule in middle class circles.

But perhaps Kemble's initial distress is more telling than the stolen finery of an escaped slave. Indeed, one only has to recall that the eighteenth-century shaving practices that might have made Dick into an ersatz coutry squire might have also made him into a Yoruba prince. The story of African hair in America is often mysterious, obscured by the silence of crucial voices and often by the language of the tale itself. Runaway ads, for instance, are often quite detailed; masters had no usual names for slave styles, so they could only describe what they saw: hair that was "woolly," "thick," and "high," sometimes "bushy" or "somewhat different from a Negro," shaved in places, but also "curled in locks" or combed "in the shape of a roll." Equally as often, these accounts betray surprise: to their masters, these runaways had "very remarkable" hair they could style to "great" heights, and with which they took "uncommon Pains." Neither a lexicon of admiration nor of contempt, these ads are rather an account of puzzlement. Like storms, witches, fevers, and the slaves themselves, to white Americans, African hair seemed to emerge from a mysterious region not fully understood.

The story of African hair in America is marked not only by moments of misunderstanding, but also moments of contradiction, symptoms of the larger gulf that separated black and white lives. One former slave told WPA interviewers about an ongoing argument he had with his mistress, who was also his grandmother. She insisted that what the slave had growing from his head was not "hair," it was "wool." When the slave resisted, claiming to have hair, his mistress would command him to correct himself. "Don't say 'hair,' " she'd direct him, "say 'wool.' " Elsie Clews Parsons, a white anthropologist, briefly discusses beauty practices in her study *Folk-Lore of the Sea Islands, South Carolina*, written in 1923. Under their kerchiefs, Sea Island women often wore their hair wrapped around strings. "Thereby," Parsons wrote with authority, "the hair is supposed to grow long and straight."

But in WPA interviews a former Louisiana slave named Amos Lincoln describes the same practice: "I 'member how d'gals uster dress up some Sunday," he remembered. "All week dey wear dey hair all roll up wid cotton dat dey unfol' off d'cotton boll. Sunday come dey comb dey hair out fine. . . . Dey want it nice and nat'ral curly." Another Louisiana man, Olivier Blanchard, remembered women using fish skins instead of cotton. But he, too, recalled the object being to curl rather than straighten the hair. "I think it eel fish they strip the skin off," he said, "and wrap round the hair and make it curly." Unable to imagine any other goal for such "uncommon pains," Parsons concludes that the Sea Island women wish for long, straight hair. Amos

Lincoln and Olivier Blanchard are equally able to imagine women going to trouble for that which is not attractive; they think the women wanted their hair curly in the end. We can't know exactly what the Sea Island women were thinking as they tied their hair in strings, so only one thing is utterly clear: one woman's straight is another man's curly.

This kind of cloudiness permeates African-American history in general, and the story of African hair in particular. Even the most basic vocabulary can seem opaque as it travels between white and black worlds. Former slaves remembered using handheld hackles—wooden "cards" with metal teeth used to "comb," or "card," wool before it is spun into yarn—to comb their hair on southern plantations. They referred to these as Jim Crow cards, using a name that was popularized for white audiences first in blackface minstrel shows of the 1850s and 1860s, and later in conjunction with southern segregation laws that were only dismantled one hundred years later, in the 1950s and 1960s. With cork-darkened faces, wooly wigs, and thick accents, minstrel singers promised their audience an "authentic" peek at black life through songs and jokes told in dialect. T. D. Rice, the founding father of blackface minstrelsy, claimed to have "discovered" black singing and dancing while traveling in the South. Outside a theater in Louisville, he is supposed to have spotted a slave performing for himself what was to become the anthem of the nineteenth-century minstrel show, "Jump Jim Crow," a dialect song that narrates its own jig in the chorus: "eb'ry time I wheel about/I jump Jim Crow."

Though the extreme popularity of the minstrel show might explain how the emerging character of Jim Crow, a combination of earnest fieldhand and Bojangles puppet, came to represent the black man, it is still unclear how Jim Crow came to represent the machinery of segregation. Northern abolitionists fought against the use of Jim Crow cars on northern railways as early as the 1840s, though it was not until fifty years later, after the abolition of slavery, that southern states began to implement Jim Crow laws stipulating strict racial segregation in all facets of public life. Depending on your perspective, it could be a long journey or a just a short leap from the Jim Crow comb to the Jim Crow water fountain. It seems, though, that what historian C. Vann Woodward has aptly called "the strange career of Jim Crow" might have begun in the tangled hair of overworked slaves. Jim Crow was a singer, a dancer, and the keeper of railroad cars; it seems he was also a hairdresser.

Nappy-Headed Blues

Like the songs, tales, and religion of slavery, slave hair has a legacy. American slaves were able to bequeath a host of African hairdressing practices to their progeny; these are the visible reminders that long ago, this hair made a troubled trip across the ocean. At the same time, there are other, less tangible but no less powerful signs of struggle: a tangled lexicon and a thicket of negative images. If black hair had an African history to remember and preserve, it also had an American present to overcome. The astonishment of the earliest white observers of black hair is indeed genuine surprise, but it is the surprise of the victor over the oddities of the vanquished. "Remarkable" literally means "deserving of remark," and thus implies a noticeable strangeness, an alien quality that should be discussed. So many hundreds of years ago, the slave system planted the seeds of modern beauty ideals. White people had hair, which could be lovely, shiny, even ugly, and black people had something different and inevitably less—wool, perhaps.

It shouldn't be surprising, then, that so many African Americans feel shame when discussing their hair. Over the course of the nineteenth century, as acculturation and the trappings of white society became more accessible to newly freed slaves, a grading system emerged for black hair, straighter being "better" than kinky. By the 1920s, Zora Neale Hurston was able to include accepted definitions for different grades of hair in the glossary of a sketch published in *American Mercury*, "Story in Harlem Slang." Characteristically blunt, Hurston's grading system only has room for dualities: "Bad Hair" is "Negro Hair," "Nearer My God to Thee" is "Good Hair," and "Good Hair" is "Caucasian-type hair." In her autobiography, *I Know Why the Caged Bird Sings*, Maya Angelou, singer, performer, and inaugural poet, describes her adolescent self as "[a] too big Negro girl, with nappy black hair, broad feet, and a space between her teeth that would hold a number two pencil." Her revenge on the children who teased her would be the revelation of her true identity as a fairy princess. "Wouldn't they be surprised when one day I woke out of my black ugly dream, and my real hair, which was long and blond, would take the place of the kinky mass Momma wouldn't let me straighten?"

Indeed, the grading system that equates what is generally black—kinkiness—with what is bad, making physical judgements coincide with moral assumptions, has become a stock symbol of oppression for African American essayists. Everyone from Angela Davis to Henry Louis Gates, Jr., to Alice Walker to random columnists in *Ebony* and *Jet* remembers where they fell on the scale. In grocery lines and salon chairs, women, especially, wince when they recall the pain of being told they had "nappy," "kinky," *bad* black hair. (Yes, those were the days before bad meant good.) But the children . . . the children seem to have a classification system all their own. They still grade hair with the same bold fervor, but the lines seem to have shifted. The moral imperative hasn't dissolved, bad hair is still shakily but definitely linked to bad*ness*, and yet the simple racial equation—bad=black—has blurred around the edges.

At a playground on the corner of 120th Street and St. Nicholas Avenue in Harlem, I meet Nathaniel "Papa Daddy" Rittenhour, who is surprised that someone might take his street name—Papa Daddy—to mean that he is himself the father of young children. He is not. A high school student who is studying to be a certified nurse's assistant, Nathaniel is instead something of an anthropologist. He has been studying the hair fashions of St. Nicholas Avenue for some time, and is pleased to have someone interested in his observations, despite the misgivings of his friend, Corey, who cringes when Nathaniel introduces him by name—"Aw, man, what if she's the police?" Several boys play basketball nearby as Nathaniel and a few others lean up against the brick wall of the school that flanks the playground, which is really just a yard of concrete with two basketball hoops at one end. When the players come over to the group for water, which they drink from large bottles with neon logos and then splash over their torsos, Nathaniel becomes the runway announcer, introducing their hair and evaluating it for the crowd. Benjy, a small wiry boy who is older than he looks, has managed to pass their somewhat rigid inspection. "That's about as good as it's gonna get," says Nathaniel, nodding at Benjy, whose hair is cut short and travels in shallow but distinct waves away from his face. Benjy uses S-Curl, a men's relaxer you can buy at a drugstore, and then a "do-rag," a nylon cloth that ties around the head while the hair dries in order to keep it from puffing up. Aware that he is on display, he runs home in between games and changes into a shiny black T-shirt with matching athletic pants, an outfit that makes him look like a child singer about to go on stage. He seems pleased but not surprised at Nathaniel's assessment.

Nathaniel lets out a yell of pain when another young boy comes into the playground because this boy's hair is *peasy*— it has knotted into little pea-shaped balls on his head, and between them, you can see his scalp. He, too, does not seem surprised by Nathaniel's accusation, but rather resigned, like someone who is teased often but not too hard. Nathaniel sums up this young man's situation: "Certain people can't get waves," he says, almost about to let the boy off the hook by virtue of genetic defect. "Their hair's too peasy!" He breaks into laughter and his meaning is clear—

no one is born to peas. They are the effect of a lack of style, possibly of self-neglect. You can overcome them if you really want to.

For girls, the idea of bad hair is not so easy to shrug off with a laugh. Certainly, it's far more serious than cartoon peas. "Good hair you can put up in lots of styles and it's soft," says Antoya, a Fort Greene fifth grader who is reading while she waits to have her hair styled at Niccki's Unisex Salon. She has been sitting here for over an hour now while her stylist finishes someone else's hair, and the pink tassel of her bookmark is starting to swing impatiently as she drums her feet against the bench.

Good hair is easy for her to describe, and she smiles as she tells all of the things it can do: you can wear it up, in a ponytail, or a braid; you can plait it into cornrows; or you can even wear it "out," with barrettes or a headband or even nothing in it. But bad hair is not so easily pinned down, so to speak. "Bad hair," she says slowly, "is not soft. It's not nice." She thinks for a minute, trying to find a way to sum up all the ways bad hair is bad hair. Finally, she decides that a simple opposition is best. Perhaps she worries I won't understand anything more complicated, since I have already proven myself uneducated by asking. "It's hair you can only do one thing with." Antoya's hair, which is exactly the same color as her eyes, is caught back in a pink scrunchy now, and she is waiting for her stylist to braid it in cornrows. She is proud of its versatility and, of course, its texture, which, according to Antoya, is the softness that allows her ponytail to extend several inches past its pink scrunchy and to swing when she shakes her head. I ask her if her hair is good hair. She looks toward the floor and nods.

"But who has bad hair?" I ask her. An apologetic smile turns her lips and she shrugs. She's not ready for slander yet at this stage in our relationship; unlike Nathaniel, she does not think bad hair is funny at all. "Is it the dorky girls who have bad hair?" Sadly, with a grave look, Antoya nods. "Yes," she whispers. "The dorks."

Whitney, who has just finished having her hair styled, is holding a newborn that begins to cry just as its mother settles in for her shampoo. Whitney tickles the baby's face with the curled ends of her freshly straightened hair, and the baby swings at the air, now perfectly content. Whitney is only eleven, but she is tall and very serious and holds the baby with one arm, like a pro, gently tipping her into the plush of her white sweatshirt. At her Seventh Day Adventist school in Fort Greene, the cool girls wear their hair like Whitney's—long, straight, and relaxed. In fact, after a moment of consideration, Whitney decides that this is just exactly what good hair is, hair like her own that is soft, straightened, and swings past your chin. Bad hair is hair that is "damaged, with split ends." It is hair she doesn't often see at her school, where almost all of her friends—she seems to have a lot of friends—have good hair. A grimace passes over her smooth, grave, eleven-year-old face and, like Antoya, she speaks softly when she tells me who in her world has bad hair. With sincere, deeply felt pity, she leans in close to my ear. "I see a lot of people on the street with bad hair." She whispers, I think, so the baby won't hear.

This distinction between good hair and bad hair has a long history of industrial support. As early as the 1830s and

1840s, when the numbers and buying power of free blacks was limited, certain products promised to solve the beauty problems inherent in blackness—kinky hair and black skin. Indeed, Black Skin Remover, Curl-I-Cure ("A Cure for Curls"), and sundry other remedies, including wigs, were the only products on the market aimed specifically and exclusively at black Americans. Ads vowed that Black Skin Remover, manufactured by Crane and Co., in Richmond, Virginia, "will turn the skin of a black or brown person four or five shades lighter, and a mulatto person perfectly white." Customers who purchased Crane and Co.'s Hair Straightener were assured of complete confidentiality—a discreet package, and a free container of "No Smell." And though most manufacturers of black hair products were white-owned companies, a small number of free blacks in the North, like the famous Remond sisters, abolitionists and makers of Mrs. Putnam's Medicated Hair Tonic, also participated. The Remonds' wig factory, Ladies Hair Work, was the biggest·wig factory in Massachusetts in the middle of the nineteenth century.

It was in the early decades of the twentieth century, however, that the black beauty industry really took off, with black entrepreneurs like Anthony Overton and Madame C. J. Walker leading the way. Madame Walker, suffering herself from hair trouble, was visited by a large black man in a dream. He counseled her on what would become the formula for her famous Hair Grower, which she sold in conjunction with a newly devised straightening comb and pressing oil, meant to protect the hair from the heat of the comb and also to help with the straightening process. The first black female millionaire in the United States, Madame

Walker was followed avidly by both the black and white presses. *Literary Digest* named her the "Queen of Gotham's Colored 400," and reported that the furniture in her bedroom at her Westchester estate cost forty-five hundred dollars. Even more than her competitor, Annie Turnbo Malone, who invented Poro Products, Madame Walker was celebrated as an entrepreneur and as a model for black women: an uneducated southern orphan and a widowed mother, a former washerwoman, she became a pioneer in an industry that would become a staple in the black economy.

Over one hundred thousand blacks left the South in the years before and after the first world war, most of them settling in northern cities which seemed to offer more opportunity than the rural South, but which were in truth crowded and, often, inhospitable. This was the Great Migration that spawned the Harlem Renaissance and drew the attention of white America as no other black cultural offering had before or has since. Black cultural figures like Langston Hughes, Zora Neale Hurston, and Duke Ellington seemed, for a time at least, to present America with its own best self—vibrant, creative, and racially tolerant. Although it has become a cliché, emblematic of condescension and voyeurism, for a moment white America celebrated its other half, frequenting Harlem nightclubs like Small's and the Cotton Club, which, it is true, often turned their backs on their black clientele in order to serve whites in the manner to which they had become accustomed. But when Alain Locke, Harlem's ambassador to white America, proclaimed the advent of the "New Negro" in 1925, it was more than palliative patter for anxious whites; he was voicing the hope of the moment.

In this fluid climate, where both hope and frustration were secondary to the sheer momentum of possibility, the commercial beauty industry flourished. Indeed, as a vocation and as an avocation, beauty was the perfect symbol for the Great Migration: a respectable job with a steady income, hairdressing required skill and allowed thousands of women to quit the fields and earn their way in the urban North. Madame Walker's beauty courses promised women credentials, opportunity, freedom, and mobility. Ads for Pittsburgh's Lelia College of Hair Culture, the first Walker school, boasted that their course was "Your Passport to Prosperity" and praised the Walker System as "a real opportunity for women who wish to become independent." Sensing danger, the Georgia state legislature imposed a tax on beauty salons, because they lured laborers from the fields. In Chicago, a prime destination for northbound blacks, salons rivaled eateries for the migrants' attention. In 1920, there were 119 delis in Chicago and 108 beauty shops. Without knowing it, the *New York Times* captured the dual nature of urban beauty culture during the Great Migration: there were so many beauty shops in Harlem that "the stranger gets the idea that many members of the colored race must be afflicted with baldness, or think their hair needs some sort of treatment."

It was true: Harlem had three times as many beauty salons as any other part of New York; many Harlem residents did indeed think that their hair needed "some sort of treatment"; and no doubt many were "afflicted with baldness." Dermatologists even have a name for the hair loss caused by many of those treatments—"hot-comb alopecia" in the vernacular, "follicular degeneration syndrome" in medical terms. What became true in the 1920s remains true today: a fashionable new appearance became the watchword for urban success and upward mobility, and for many women, this meant straightening their hair. Settlement workers, teachers, and newspaper editors worked to improve the appearance of the newly arrived, and urban memoirs painfully rehearse the humiliation of being counseled on grooming, hygiene, and fashion. This was an experience that migrant blacks shared with Jewish and Italian immigrants. African-American magazines often urged readers not to send their children to school with their hair wrapped in strings since it evoked an image of country folkways instead of urban sophistication. The *Saturday Evening Post* noted the connection between the burgeoning beauty industry and the social and economic aspirations of the newly arrived urban migrants. "The first thing every Negro girl does when she comes from the South is to have her hair straightened." The first thing every Jewish woman did when she came from Poland was remove her wig.

When Jews, Italians, and other sources of cheap labor joined the army, graduated to white collar work, or returned to Europe at the start of the war, urban manufacturers began recruiting black workers in the South, luring them with free train tickets and promises of success. At the same time, immigrant neighborhoods like Harlem experienced a similar influx: Jews and Italians slowly moved out, making their way to the suburbs or back to Italy, and African Americans moved in. For the first three decades of this century, Harlem was a melange of cultures, albeit an often tense and periodically violent one. The hair industry reflected (indeed, it still does) this strained but real connection among Harlem's three main ethnic groups—blacks, Jews, and Italians. Although blacks often ran African-American beauty shops, they rarely owned the buildings that housed them. And though black hair care companies like Madame Walker's consistently outsold white-owned companies like Golden Brown, the wig industry, which was also an important resource for black beauty products, was dominated by Jewish and Italian wig manufacturers and hair importers. But blacks and Jews shared a beauty handicap, for which black companies had a solution. In an ad in the enormously popular Yiddish-language daily the *Forward*, Madame Walker sounded the alarm. "Froien!" the ad screams in Yiddish, "here is the answer to your questions about beauty! We use modern techniques to treat dry, hard and *gekreiselte* hair." *Gekreiselte* means kinky in Yiddish.

And yet, for all their popularity, beauty products like hair straighteners and skin bleaches were not universally accepted. The debate about the propriety of altering one's appearance so distinctly is as old as the products themselves. Even before the Civil War made freedom and prosperity a legal possibility, black leaders cautioned their peers against trying to emulate whites in appearance. Just as social scientists were beginning to adapt Darwinism to the logic of racial preference, black writers like Martin Freeman counseled pride and perseverance. At the same time, he ridiculed efforts to eradicate African features, especially the "straightening process" through which kinky hair is "oiled and pulled, twisted up, tied down, sleeked over, and pressed under . . ." The rapidly expanding African-American press of the 1920s provided fuel and a forum for the debate. While columnists railed against the racist assumptions of the beauty industry, cosmetic and toiletry firms bought between thirty and forty percent of the ad space sold by black papers. Even activist newspapers like Marcus Garvey's *Negro World* could not resist the revenue offered by beauty ads.

Reacting in part to charges of racial denigration, and in part to an increasingly public and articulate racial pride, cosmetic companies began to use celebratory images of African beauty in the 1920s. Cleopatra became the stock symbol of female African majesty, and *Egyptian*, *Creole*, and *Mediterranean* became code words for black but not too black, a blackness of which one could be proud. Beauty messages of the 1920s were as mixed as they are today: optimism, pride, and possibility, but also confusion, chaos, and contradiction. Hortense Powdermaker, another northern anthropologist who studied the South in the 1920s, noted how very important it was to blacks of Cottonville, Mississippi, a pseudonymous town in the Yazoo Delta, to be neither too dark nor too light. "To make a 'good' marriage means to marry 'light,' " noticed Powdermaker, though for those who were themselves "very dark," the prospect of a light-skinned mate was often intimidating. One light-skinned woman who had moved to Cottonville from a nearby city explained why a light-skinned mate was essential to her: " 'Who,' she asks with a shudder and a laugh, 'would want to have a black-skinned baby with kinky hair?' "

Such ambivalence seems to be built into the language of

the industry, lending it a slightly sinister, cagey tone. When hair that has been straightened with a hot comb and pressing oil gets wet, it is said to "go" or "turn back," as if it had been asked to hold an impossible pose or keep an impossible promise. Black women who wear their hair straightened in this way are devoted to the sun, and fear the rain like Superman fears kryptonite. Turned by fashion into mad scientists, they await the undoing of their chemical experiments by the most essential of elements, water. In the 1930s and 1940s, black musicians and their followers popularized a permanent chemical straightening process now honed and refined and called the relaxer. Back then it was called a conk, a descriptive, onomatopoetic name that bespeaks a friendly sort of violence, a rap on the head that produces an instant welt when Bugs Bunny does it to Daffy Duck. No one can say for certain where the term comes from: it might have originated with a New York barber named William Hart who called his popular concoction Kink No More; some remember that Kink made Conk by a simple vowel substitution—*o* replaced *i*. Others think it came from another preparation, Kongolene Knocks Kinks, the *g* being that hard, immigrant sort of *g* that might as well be a *k*. Conk-o-lene, some say.

Whatever its origin, the consonance of the acronym stutters violently. Quickly, too easily, Kongolene Knocks Kinks became KKK, KKK became conk, and other things, too. Henry Louis Gates, Jr., remembers his father's KKK: Knotty, Kinky, and Kan't-comby. A stunned New York barber thought of something else when a client sat back in his chair and told him to slap three Ks on his head. He thought of the picture he'd seen recently of Alexander

Johnson, a black Texan kidnapped and tortured by the Ku Klux Klan. As a way of reminding him of the order of things, who he was and who they were, they'd branded his forehead straight across with their three Ks.

"Free at Last"

Like other apocryphal tales, hair-straightening stories are traumatic, if triumphant, legends. All at once, they substantiate and deflate the hubris of modern science: we now know that when we apply lye—sodium hydrochloride, what we might use to make soap, as in Lysol—to human hair, it permanently alters the molecular structure of the hair. In lay terms, what was curly suddenly goes straight. We also know that it can hurt like hell. When lye is left long enough on the scalp, it starts to burn. Left longer, it does burn. The usual story is a child's: someone left the relaxer in too long, and soon the kid was crying, screaming. Spike Lee told Malcolm X's version, with a twist: when the burning starts and the pipes don't work, a desperate Malcolm goes for the only water in the house. The police come to arrest Malcolm just as he sticks his head in the toilet; obviously, he has hit rock bottom in every sense. (In *The Autobiography of Malcolm X*, the toilet incident happens long before Malcolm is arrested for robbery. He is visiting his family in Michigan, where the pipes aren't reliable enough for big city conks.)

Annu Prestonia, owner of Khamit Kinks, a braiding salon in Atlanta and New York, associates her hair-straightening trauma with her family's move from Virginia to New York.

Not wanting to cost her mother more money than was absolutely necessary, Annu thought she could make sure her relaxer lasted longer than usual. "I didn't tell them it was burning," she remembers, and the relaxer began to eat away at her hair and scalp. She stood it for as long as she could, but a lot of her hair didn't survive. "Whatever didn't break off had to be cut off." This is the thirty-year-old story Annu remembers when she sits down to talk about her salon and how she got started doing braids. It is the reason she used a pressing comb in high school, even though it meant she had to re-press (repress?) her hair daily to keep up her style. And, it is the memory that guided her, like a Biblical parable, to her decision to wear her own hair in braids and then, ultimately, to make braids her business. She was surprised, then, how popular her short, short hair was. "They thought I was ahead of my time," she says of her schoolmates and teachers, many of whom followed suit and had their hair cut short. "I remember the devastation of being bald-headed."

Despite its rhetoric of longevity and languor, straightening one's hair with chemicals is neither permanent nor relaxing. Even though today's formulas are much gentler than Malcolm Little's potato-lye conk, over time, treatments often take their toll on the hair, causing it to break off or fall out, or both. The hair that has been treated won't "go back" like hair that has been straightened with a hot comb, but new hair grows in curly, so the process has to be repeated every four to six weeks. It is almost impossible to keep all of your hair straight all of the time: there's the regrowth, the telltale "nappy edges" Ntozake Shange wrote about, and there's the "kitchen," the fast-growing hair at the back of the neck that is hard to reach with a pressing comb. Henry Louis Gates, Jr., thinks of it as a metaphor for the resilient souls of black folks. It is an expression of an inner appetite that won't change no matter how straight, or white, the rest of you becomes: "Neither God nor woman nor Sammy Davis, Jr., could straighten the kitchen," he writes. "[It] was permanent, irredeemable, irresistible kink." For Nathaniel and his friends at the St. Nicholas Avenue playground, a nappy kitchen means that it's time for a girl to go to the beauty parlor. They call those curly kitchen hairs "buckshots," and though they're not as bad as peas, they're not good, either. Nathaniel supports the out-of-sight, out-of-mind approach to buckshots. "Some girls shave it off," he says approvingly.

A rejection of the cost, pain, and racial implications of chemical relaxers and perms, the Afro of the 1960s celebrated kink, a hair texture that many considered uniquely African. By association, it celebrated anything that opposed white power and intransigence, and figures now as a visual icon that captures all of the turmoil, hope, and anger of those years. Both literally and figuratively, the Afro lent stature to those who wore it, making it the perfect expression of black pride and power. In her autobiography, activist Assata Shakur echoed Martin Luther King when she remembered her first Afro: she cut the perm out of her hair, washed out the last of the chemicals, and finally, she wrote, her hair was "free at last."

Although for many the Afro was a hairstyle like any other, for Black Panther activists like Angela Davis, it was the stylistic implementation of a political commitment. At a European conference she attended as a young student, Davis's hairstyle made her immediately recognizable as a sympathizer with the black power movement. Many years later, at her infamous California trial, one of the government's witnesses claimed to recognize Davis as a former customer at his filling station. He knew it was her, he said, because of her light complexion and her Afro.

As a protest against the monotonous beauty standards of white America, the Afro was a success, linked forever in our minds with the raised-fist salute of men in black turtlenecks. And as a style, too, the Afro traveled far. Nearly everyone old enough to remember disco remembers the shape of their 'fro and the battle with their parents to let them wear their hair high and mighty. For many, the Afro was not just a rejection of a white aesthetic, it was a rebellion against parental authority. Naydene, a systems analyst I meet at Khamit Kinks on a Saturday afternoon, had long, much-admired hair when she was in elementary school in Newark, New Jersey. No one else in her family had such "good" hair, and Naydene's mother adamantly rejected her daughter's desire to wear it short. One Saturday afternoon, Naydene walked to a barber shop in her neighborhood and told the surprised barber, "Cut it."

"I was saying I wanted my independence," she remembers. She wanted a big Afro, not the long doll's hair her mother thought she should have. After cutting it, she tried to cultivate the halo of hair worn by her favorite pop stars. But in the end, her hair was too straight to hold the Jackson Five Afro she wanted. It was, in fact, too "good."

Many recall the Afro with humor, as if its power was a

matter of adolescent pretense, a briefly held posture of defiance. And, indeed, for a style that fancied itself the antidote to centuries of oppression, the Afro's historical moment was short-lived. By the late 1970s, it was gone, replaced by the low-riding and much-maligned Jheri curl. Some think that the Afro died by its own accord, crushed under its own excessive weight, so to speak. At first, Roxanne, a fashion designer and makeup artist who grew up in East New York, sparkles when she describes her childhood Afro. "We were Muslim, and couldn't press our hair," says Roxanne, whose green eye shadow stretches past her carefully arched brows. Her voice booms and she seems ready to speak for everyone gathered at Niccki's Unisex in Fort Greene this Friday afternoon, even though she is the only one in the group who has just stopped in to chat. She's had her short curly hair cut recently, and doesn't need anything but company today. As a small child, she wore her hair in pineapple braids—a single cornrow that spirals around the head and finishes in a little knot at the top. It was a child's style with adult meaning. "We were supposed to remain the way we came," she says.

Later, she wore a real Afro. "You would wash it, grease it with . . . Afro-Sheen." She and Lisha, an administrator at Bankers Trust, say this in unison, with a laugh, as if they are recalling an old but slightly embarrassing friend from high school. "Then you'd braid it, while it was still damp, and roll it. The next morning, you'd unleash the braids. It was *beautiful,*" Roxanne says, shaking her head at the memory. Her eyes slightly glazed, Lisha begins shaking her head, too, her long face smiling at the audacity of her preadolescent self. She's come to Niccki's this afternoon to get her hair, which she dismisses as a "mess," "taken care of." A moment later, though, she has gone from fond disbelief to wry surprise. She is thinking of Roxanne's routine. "There was nothing easy about that Afro," she says.

Contrary to expectation, the Afro never made a real comeback. Today's ubiquitous short men's styles may indeed be more "natural" than the conk, but they resemble a fifties buzz cut more than they do the Afro. The braided styles of the 1990s are a different matter. In theory, at least, they owe a considerable debt to Afro ideology. They have inherited the mantle of afrocentricity and all its implications: like the Afro, they are touted as a "natural" alternative to chemicals, and an African response to the strictures of white American beauty standards. Unlike the Afro, braids have a highly visible place in African history; their authenticity makes them a popular and perhaps less threatening expression of cultural solidarity.

Annu Prestonia remembers the exact moment when braided styles went mainstream. It was in 1992, after an *Essence* magazine beauty article featured a style known as goddess braids, in which one or two thick braids are worn pinned up. Her braiding salon, Khamit Kinks, had provided the styling for the shot, and Prestonia's business suddenly took off. Since then, Prestonia has gone from a small shop in Brooklyn to a multichair TriBeCa salon with blond wood floors, copper lamp shades, and laminated menus from which her customers order lunch. "Goddess braids were a very sophisticated style," Prestonia recalls. "It wasn't hanging down and didn't need to be manipulated." More important, it didn't seem too extreme or too African. "Black people had been brainwashed. When they thought of Africa, they saw Tarzan and little pygmies who ate white folks," Prestonia says, laughing. But as goddess braids and other styles became more popular, a stylistic affiliation with African culture became easier for blacks. With exposure, and the example of stars and beauty queens, braided styles became widely accepted.

Andrea Barton-Reeves, a Manhattan attorney, has worn her hair in braids for the past five years. Every three months, she returns to Khamit Kinks, where she spends an evening and then an entire Saturday having her shoulder-length braids removed and then put back in. Because Andrea's own hair is thick and she wears her braids quite long, with synthetic hair forming the length of the braid, it takes two braiders eight hours to finish her style; on average, this costs her four hundred dollars a visit. In the early 1980s, she remembers, braids were much more of a political statement than they are now. "It meant you weren't willing to assimilate," says Andrea. Part of Andrea's decision to wear her hair in braids is also politically motivated. "I'm moving away from a form of assimilation that I thought my relaxed hair represented. I think a lot of our people are tired of manipulating their bodies and their hair for a culture that won't accept them anyway." But, like most of her nineties peers, who seem less militant, perhaps less confident, than their 1960s counterparts, Andrea is also motivated by style. Her college Afro was a statement of pride and commitment, but it was also a bore. "It looked the same every day," says Andrea, her head nodding slightly as the stylists, Thema and Deana, weave long strands of synthetic hair onto her own. "I like variety." With her hair in braids, she can wear different styles. "It's as if it was relaxed," she says, "but it's not."

Braided hair might share a certain versatility with relaxed hair, but they are not completely interchangeable. Aware that a number of women on the east coast have been fired from their jobs in the past fifteen years for wearing their hair in braids, Andrea approached her boss when she first wanted to braid her hair. She was working at an insurance company then, and did not want to spark controversy or to suddenly become a radical, threatening presence. "I couldn't just pretend that it was just another hairstyle," she says. "It was unfortunate, but I knew that was the reality." When she first began working for the midtown law firm she is with now, people stared at her hair. She had interviewed for the job with her braids, and saw no reason to take them out when she began working there. Her colleagues are used to her style now, and are less curious, but Andrea still feels out of sync. She wonders if it is the technology of the braids that makes them mysterious to her white peers. "I don't think the people I work with understand that my hair doesn't grow on my head like theirs does," she says, irony rounding out her even voice.

Andrea's mother also thought her daughter's choices contrary and inexplicable. In her sixties now, Andrea's mother still wears her hair relaxed and curled in a style that, according to Andrea, bespeaks a deep-rooted beauty conservatism. Guyanese immigrants who have lived in the United States for forty years, Andrea's parents have retained what Andrea considers a European attitude toward hair. For them, braids are "attractive, but inappropriate," in part because the braiding industry is so newly established. "Braids are what was done in other peoples' kitchens," explains Andrea. Her mother pleads with her to return to her relaxed style. "She says, 'You don't have to do that. Your father and I can afford to send you to the beauty parlor.' "

As both an expression of African heritage and a function of American pragmatism, braid styles worn here in the United States occupy a roomy middle ground. The practice of braiding has been handed down from Africa, but often, the silhouette is unmistakably white—a short bob or even a Dorothy Hamill wedge. If braiding were a mode of communication, one might say that the language is African, but the syntax is white European, precise and angled. In the pantheon of styles popular today, "locks" perform a multicultural improvisation similar to that of braided styles. Borrowing both inspiration and technique from the Jamaican Rastafarian movement, and by extension, from African styles, today's locks—yesterday's *dread*locks, or dreads—are also a statement of aesthetic independence and a rejection of beauty standards that critique the texture of black hair. But whereas Rastafarian hair logic derived from a strict reading of the biblical oath of the Nazarenes, which requires adherents to let their hair grow, those who wear locks in the late 1990s generally distance themselves from any religious connection to Rastafarianism. Nor have they generally adopted Rastafarian political ideology, which categorically rejected the institutions of white colonialism and sought redemption through return to an independent Africa. Like braids, locks have become a symbol of an amorphous, though truly felt, allegiance with African culture, and a celebration of a uniquely black aesthetic.

Hence, the loss of the *dread* prefix and its negative connotations. Today's rhetoric stresses the natural and organic, almost therapeutic, essence of locks. Those who wear them say: this is what is natural, pure, and good, to let your hair grow its curly way without chemical interference. By twisting it, the generally accepted technique for starting and maintaining locks, the stylist is helping the curl "do what it wants to do," curl even tighter around itself. Because hair can take anywhere from three to six months to begin to "lock"—that is, for the hair to start to wrap around itself by itself—locking is seen as a process that requires commitment. It is an intense hairstyle that demands patience, cultivation, and love. Swinging between Goldie and Dread, locks get momentum from their own malleable grammar: to aspire to locks is to yearn *to lock*, to place and train the hair. It is a process that implies permanence, struggle, and ultimately, détente—what is locked in is contained, safe and secure. A contradictory logic, to be sure, but also an inspiration.

Nathaniel's buddy Corey, who claims to be afraid that I am somehow affiliated with the police, wears his hair in short, feisty locks that bump against each other when he moves. He is a freshman at Hunter College, and thinks that perhaps he will study to become a physical therapist. I understand that his slightly defensive fear of police is just that—the slightly defensive, reflexive fear of someone who grew up on the southern edge of West Harlem, where the life expectancy of a black male is the same as it is in Bangladesh. After a brief perusal of my notebook, he is willing to tell me about his hair. "Locks," he says, "are a symbol of righteousness and knowledge of self." Does he feel righteous and know himself? "Hell, yeah."

"More Money Than a Taxi Driver"

Harlem's 125th Street has its own soundtrack; it is the beat that emanates from crowded storefronts, from vendors' tables set up on the sidewalk, from handheld stereos carried along by youths who cannot bear to leave their music at home. In the 1920s, the street was dominated by Jewish merchants, and the faded signs—Blumstein's—still hover above what has become an African-American and Latino thoroughfare, where merchants hawk airbrushed portraits of Malcolm X on red, yellow, and green T-shirts. On every block there is another sign promising African braids, authentic, beautiful, cheap. All over Harlem, there are these ghostly emanations: huge *shuls* consecrated as churches, their names eerie reminders of a different time—La Sinogoga Baptista—and large *mezuzahs* marking the doorways of random storefronts, the protective hallmarks of absent owners who find it best to be invisible.

The hair trade on 125th Street is brisk business: groups of African women, buttoned against the cold in colorful windbreakers, gather in front of tiny braiding salons, passing out business cards stamped with their pictures and the names of styles they can create with a little time and some synthetic hair: bouffruttu, Senegalese twists, Cassamas braids. Their low-pitched queries recall different days and different corners, where instead of "Braids, Miss?" one heard, "Smoke?

'Shroom? Need a smoke?" Here, drugstores double as beauty supply shops, with wig counters and packages of synthetic hair tucked in the back where a pharmacy counter used to be. Hand-painted signs hawk "100% Human Hair," and at places like the Hair Station and Mona Hair Supply, both owned by Koreans, you get almost nothing but: the walls are lined with unattached wefts, wigs, and bluntly cut-off ponytails in an array of textures and colors. Small markers alert the customer to the possibilities—Body Wavey, Kinky Straight, Caucasian Straight. You can buy black, blue, red, and brown, yellow, green, and purple hair. Because almost all of this hair began its life black, on the head of an Asian woman—probably Chinese, perhaps Indonesian or Thai—the lighter it is, the more it costs. The 125th Street hair business might cater to African Americans, but it certainly doesn't belong to them.

The tensions that mark this business are tiny fissures, keenly felt and complicated by market limitations of supply, demand, and race. At Adorable Hair Do, one of the largest "manufacturers" of human hair in the business, the Teitelbaum family are happy to show me their processing room, the silver tanks and blue barrels where raw hair imported from Asia and Europe is given the colors and textures of today's market. Gary Teitelbaum, one of the owners, takes a raw ponytail from a box and lets me feel its heft; it must weigh three or four pounds. It is a severed limb, eerily preserved. Asian women, he tells me, eat things that make hair grow. Gary's uncle's father, Isidore Rosen, started Adorable back in the 1910s, making wigs and hairpieces for the theatrical trade, and also for urbanizing blacks. In 1946 he developed a process for making wefts with sewing machines, eliminating the necessity of hand-tying every wig and almost putting himself out of business. He was one of the first to move his wig-making factory to Asia in the 1960s, where labor and hair were both cheap and plentiful, but by the 1970s the competition had caught on and Adorable had abandoned wigs in order to concentrate on hair—importing it, processing it, selling it for weaves, braids, and the hand-tied wigs made by others.

Back in the beginning, Adorable was in the heart of the hair district, above the Baby Grand Nightclub on 125th Street in Harlem. Now the Adorable showrooms and offices are in the margins of the fashion district, on a side street in the west twenties. This migration, and all that it implies, makes the Teitelbaums uncomfortable. The last time they spoke to a journalist—Lisa Jones of the *Village Voice*—they came off sounding like rich white businessmen exploiting the hang-ups of poor blacks. "That's just not the case," says Gary, whose beard makes him seem even more earnest than he is. "This business is benevolent in ways that people don't see." Next to him, on the wall, a child's Happy Easter drawing projects pink-marker happiness into the crowded, work-filled room. A woman enters and climbs through the stacks of papers and ledgers to find her purse. She is headed out the door, but Gary stops her. "This is my wife, Noreen," he says, introducing her to me, the journalist whom he has trusted in spite of himself. Noreen is African American and has very long auburn hair. She leaves before I figure out if it is hers.

Gary Teitelbaum understands the social and economic divergences that led his family from Harlem but kept his customers there. He understands, and though quietly defensive, acknowledges the irony of a Jew processing Asian hair to sell to a market that is mainly black. Since there is a language barrier and a tradition of defensive reticence, it is hard to tell if the Korean merchants, who are the most visible hair vendors on 125th Street, are as self-conscious about their place in this economic tangle. Tensions flare and flash, but only for brief public seconds.

Alex, an African American who has worked at the Hair Station for twelve years now, admits that the hair hanging on the walls is Asian hair, processed in the basement of the 125th Street store, but "what we do, how we do it, that's a *secret.*" While we speak, his Korean boss abandons the soap operas she is watching at the back of the store and offers to help two women who have come in to buy hair and are having trouble deciding what they want. But her English is not up to the task, and soon she calls for help. "Alex!" The surgical tape that covers a cut on her forehead buckles as she smiles, apologizing already. One of the customers, exasperated, speaks first. "I *asked* her . . ." Alex clears up the problem and passes the hair they have decided to buy to his boss, who rings up the purchase, bags the hair, and hands it back to Alex. He then gives it to the customer. The women look at each other, offended by this inexplicable ritual, the apparent unwillingness of the Korean woman to face her black customers. "What?" one asks the other. "She doesn't want to touch you?"

The mainstay of this Harlem hair economy, African braiding practices, taught by every mother to every daughter, have become a mythical passport to prosperity for African immigrants. Those planning to cross the ocean to join husbands, fathers, and brothers, many of whom drive cabs or work as security guards, pass the word on: I hear in America, if you can braid hair, you can get . . . a watch, a television, a car . . . But, like most immigrant myths, the story fades on this side of the ocean. It is possible to make money braiding hair, but competition and new licensing requirements are making it harder. Most braiders are here illegally, and are hobbled by the familiar problems of deracination—no English, no rights, no clout. Many have little education and no other skills.

"Braiding is the only way they can survive," says Amminata Sy Keneme, a bilingual counselor at the African Services Committee who braided hair herself after a United Nations fellowship ended and left her to rely on her hands for work. She estimates that seventy-five percent of African immigrants rely on braiding to eat. For most beginners, braiding in a salon is the easiest and fastest way to get started, though the fixed salary can be limiting: many times, the braider will complete four or five heads a day, at $100–$120 per head, but only receive $150–$180 per week. Braiders can rent a chair in a shop for about a hundred dollars a week, but this can be risky business, especially if you have no established clientele.

Hence, the 125th Street hustle. One Guinean woman I meet on the corner of Adam Clayton Powell Boulevard and 125th pays six thousand dollars a month to rent the long, narrow second-floor space that she and her five partners, in a gesture of extreme pragmatism, have named 125th African Hair Braiding. With the familiar plaintive whisper, "Want braids?" she stands on the street with three other women, handing out cards to those who pass by in the Saturday morning rush. All four women have their hair hidden under caps; their advertisements are magazine pictures pasted to a freestanding sandwich board. Upstairs, chairs that rent for two hundred dollars a month are occupied by customers who sit and listen to African music, their heads tipped back with the pull of the weave. Around their feet are bunches of discarded synthetic hair, a dark, indifferent carpet hiding dirty gray linoleum. With the four to eight hundred dollars a week she makes from braiding (she won't say what she makes on rent), she is proof of Amminata Sy Keneme's less-than-encouraging prediction: "If you have a good salon, you'll make more money than a taxi driver."

"Had it not been for them, I might have been a millionaire by now," says Annu Prestonia of the influx of African braiders, many of whom produce elaborate styles for less than half the price she charges at Khamit Kinks. Very few, she estimates, are true professional braiders, and very few do a good job. Their styles "look like a rug," she says. "The hairline is naturally fine, but they make it thick, with lots of braids close to the forehead. In Africa, nobody would get their hair done by them." Clumsy, thick, and unprofessional is her final assessment; you get what you pay for.

She and other salon owners are looking to the state to regulate braiding practices just as they do other salon services. Since 1993, New York State has required that anyone braiding hair receive a natural hair care license—a license that allows one to cut, braid, and lock hair, but not to administer chemicals like relaxers or colorants—but there is no enforcement of the law and relatively few practitioners have bothered to comply. As of March, 1998, only 310 natural hair care licenses have been issued in New York State. In part, this is because no large body of complaints has been issued against braiding establishments, unlike, for instance, nail salons, where unsanitary practices have led to widespread nail fungus problems. In part, however, it is also because current licensing requirements are out of sync with the realities of the profession and its training grounds. A full cosmetology license requires one thousand hours of study, usually in a course that costs between five and seven thousand dollars. A natural hair care license requires nine hundred hours of study, and so far, few schools have found it a feasible course of study. Most braiders remain unlicensed; most beauty students decide to go for one hundred more hours and get a full license.

For Annu and Diane Bailey, one of the chief lobbyists behind the decision to license natural hair care providers, the economic and legal issues are infused with cultural pride. Bailey, owner of Tendrils, a natural hair care salon in Fort Greene, maintains that without state-recognized standards, natural hair care practitioners will never receive the professional respect they deserve. Without professional recognition, she wonders, "How can you get a loan from a bank, or for a car?" At times, Bailey, who has a deep, resonant voice and hands that help her make her point, sounds like a latter-day Booker T. Washington. Braiding is indeed an art, she concedes, but in modern-day America, it is also an industry, one often practiced in seedy, unsanitary conditions. In short, it is a profession in need of some good, old-fashioned nineteenth-century "uplift."

A system of education, regulation, and licensing would ultimately "empower the community," she contends, by preserving techniques, commanding respect, and cultivating awareness. "Anyone who is touching another human body should have guidelines to mandate what they can and cannot do," she says adamantly. Preserving African tradition is also an important goal for the proponents of the licensing; Bailey and her colleagues also want to be sure that regulation does not fall to an alien or hostile force. "We want to keep it ours," says Bailey. "We want to make it clear that this is not Asian or European—it's African." Aware that these regulations, if enforced, will hit African immigrants the hardest, Bailey believes in the long-term benefits of harsh medicine. "African immigrants are being used and abused. I want them to be economically empowered as well. We're all the same."

But not everyone agrees that licensing is the way to protect African traditions or African immigrants. Taalib Din-Uqdah, a co-owner of Cornrows and Co., a natural hair salon in Washington, D.C., and the executive director of the American Hair Braiders and Natural Hair Care Association, considers the push for state licensing a sinister collaboration between the cosmetology lobby and white government. Over the eighteen years that Uqdah and his wife and business partner, Pamela Farrel, have operated their salon, African braids have become both popular styles and big business. In 1986, there were three other braiding salons in the Washington, D.C., area; now, there are thirty-six in D.C. proper, and, Uqdah estimates, between seventy-five and eighty within a forty-five-mile radius. For Uqdah, this trend toward natural hairstyles has all of the qualities of a religious revival. "There's a spirit moving around that's making people go back to their natural hair," says Uqdah, his voice a raspy preacher's roar over the phone. "This is God-inspired!"

And if the revival of traditional African styles is the good work of the Lord, the licensing lobby is the agency of the devil. Uqdah, who was once a proponent of state licensure, speaks with the bitter fervor of an apostate who has seen the light. "The people in this business are so cunning, they don't want to let anything associated with Africa come into play," he says, pitting white cosmetologists against African immigrants and African traditions. And what about those like Diane Bailey, who consider licensure the best way to preserve African traditions? "This is a classic case of someone who was once oppressed starting to oppress people," rails Uqdah. "They need to be ashamed and embarrassed!"

Indeed, the general attitude of the cosmetology establishment is, to say the least, less than Afro-centric. Beauty schools in the New York area teach relaxing and straightening techniques, but they do not incorporate natural hairstyling practices into their curricula unless there is extra time. Most of the African-American hairstylists I spoke with remember straight-haired, not curly-haired, mannequins in their classes. In classic beauty textbooks, like those published by Milady, one of the major beauty text publishers, African hair is characterized as "overcurly" or "excessively curly," a pathological deviation from the straight white norm that can be "treated" only by the trained professional. Uqdah sees licensing as a parallel process, in which black practitioners will be forced to adapt African practices to white beauty standards. "Cosmetologists like to define everything," he growls. The African members of Uqdah's coalition are frightened by the legal hurdles of the licensing process and bewildered by the bureaucratic interference. "They ask me, 'How can this be illegal in a country that represents freedom? You can have sex with anyone, you can do anything . . . but don't braid hair?' Emergency medical technicians train for less than two hundred hours . . . but braiding hair takes nine hundred?" Like New York's, D.C.'s licensing requirements have proven easier to effect than to enforce. According to Uqdah, "They haven't issued a license yet."

Mr. Uqdah and I speak for several hours on the phone; he is in his office in Washington and I am in my living room in New York City. We start talking in the pale light of an afternoon in early spring, but when we finish it is dark night and I haven't bothered to switch on the lights. Though he senses he has found a sympathetic ear, Uqdah's voice stretches across the wires, tense and urgent. We talk about the hair business, about who markets what to whom and how it sells, about how Koreans have a "lock" on the raw hair business, but it is the Jews who process it best, about how there's only one African-American company that sells Asian hair to blacks, and they're in St. Louis.

But of course, that's not really it: we're not talking about silverware or napkins or even paper plates. This isn't what we eat or eat from, it's how we look and that suddenly seems much more important. We're talking about an industry that contains and is contained by black identity, and yet is never fully managed by the black economy and has never resolved its struggle with white beauty standards. One might shrug and point to the place in the economics textbook that explains why this is so, but neither Uqdah nor I are in that kind of mood. Perhaps this is why I haven't turned on the lights.

Eventually, I come full circle. I think that braids and weaves are more than just expressions of an African aesthetic, a stylistic atavism to be revived and celebrated. They are the ghostly handiwork of the trickster, Bre'r Rabbit's joke on America, where Goldilocks and Rapunzel are always blond, a mysterious art that stretches short curly hair long and straight. Annu Prestonia worries about the ecology of synthetic hair. "When they dig us up two thousand years from now," she says, "that hair's going to be sitting right there waiting—just like it was." Another woman, a teacher at a girls school in New Jersey, looks on in alarm as her students get new weaves every week. "They're always wearing the hair they wish they had," she says, twisting one of her locks as her eyes cloud with concern. This woman laughs when she tells the story of a white colleague, who saw her chin-length locks and assumed she was not American. "I thought you were from Ghana," the woman said. "No," she told her, "I'm from Maplewood, New Jersey."

By the end of every proper trickster tale, meaning is skewed and the order of things, once so carefully stacked, will list dangerously to one side if it doesn't come crashing down. Tasha, a stylist at Niccki's salon in Fort Greene, is considering the good/bad hair question as she attaches a bone-straight weave to her customer's angular head. "I think your hair is bad hair," she says to me, her face completely sober. "People say your texture is good hair, but it's bad hair to me. It's hard to deal with. You can't do anything with it." The heat starts at the back of my neck and creeps into my cheeks. I know it is not an insult. It is, rather, a simple assessment of possibilities: my hair is kinky, too frizzy ever to be smooth and long and what I wished for as a child, but obviously not kinky enough to lock or hold braids properly. Later, I will blink back tears of relief when a black stylist touches my head and says, "Ooh—it's nappy back here," but now I'm feeling stung, rebuked. I have bad hair.

Tasha, absorbed in her task, has no idea that I have taken her words to heart. Her thoughts have moved on. "There are things more important than hair," she says, whistling. "Like what?" I'm troubled and can't even imagine what she means. What could be more important than hair? Her hand drops over her belly, which swells stoutly over her legs, and she answers with a patient smile. "Babies."

Four

Clear and Smooth as a Baby's

> And, I, stepping from this skin
> Of old bandages, boredoms, old faces
> Step to you from the black car of Lethe,
> Pure as a baby.
>
> —Sylvia Plath, "Getting There"

Beeswax, $23, Lower Leg

In deference to the military hero of the Republic, Scipio Africanus, who subdued Carthage with a blockade and made "Africa" a Roman outpost, Roman men visited their *tonsors,* or barbers, daily to have their cheeks and chins scraped free of hair. Most tonsors wielded iron razors—*novaculae*—which were notoriously difficult to sharpen, but perhaps more efficient and effective than depilatories concocted by one's *ornatrix*, the lucky slave devoted to the rich man's toilet. Part peeling plaster, part corrosive solution, Roman depilatories were an eerie collection of ingredients. For instance: resin, pitch, and ivy gum, mixed with "ass's fat, she-goat's gall, bat blood, and powdered viper." It's no wonder, then, that Caesar, fearing a sharp blade against his naked throat as well as the corrosive power of bat blood, declined the depilatory aid of Roman apothecaries, preferring instead that his ornatrix pluck his beard, hair by hair. Unlike some of his citizen counterparts, Caesar was never, as far as we know, refused his seat in the senate because of unsightly stubble; nor was he killed by the knowing blade of his tonsor. He died by the hands of his friends and former allies, presumably with cheeks as clear and smooth as a baby's.

Had Caesar been able to choose from a wider range of depilatory options, he might at least have spent less time bent to the tweezer. Today's plasters—semiliquid substances that harden around hairs and, when peeled away, pull hair out by the roots—are both simpler and more sophisticated than the Romans' pitch-and-ivy gum. Seeking long-term results and also to offset the attendant discomfort of ripping hair out of its roots, modern salons depilate with honey, beeswax, and tea-tree resin. They import purple bikini wax from Australia, where estheticians have discovered a way to "shrink-wrap" the hair, so that the wax doesn't pull on the skin. They powder first, soothe with chamomile and witch hazel, and offer copious aftercare advice: *lotion, cold water, warm water, no sun, rest, buy this potion!* Each salon maintains that their method is the sure-fire breeze, the one that grabs the hair the best and hurts the least.

Wearing a white coat, bobby socks, and rectangular black-rimmed glasses, Lea stands over two battered aluminum pots of melted beeswax set on a roller cart in the front of the wax room at Madelaine, a beauty spa on the Upper West Side of Manhattan. For the most part, Lea is uninterested in newfangled ways of soothing the skin or priming the follicles. She believes in beeswax, which she imports from Israel and France, and which she cooks on the stove in a tiny room next door, adding only "a secret" as it melts down. Before she cooks it, the solid chunks of beeswax, piled under sheets beneath the waxing tables and in the closet, have a greenish, barklike cast to them—their surface is waxy and gritty all at once—but melted, the wax is brown, the color of dense caramel. Drizzled pieces stick to the black-and-white tiled floor, and to your feet as you walk back to the dressing room, where women in their underwear wait for one of the two stretcherlike tables in Lea's room to open up. I guess at her "secret" but Lea only smiles. I go by the color, and the smell: Is it molasses? Soy sauce? Rum?

It is my turn—my first waxing!—and I'm only a little nervous. Next to me, a woman named Joan with a gros-grain headband and Calvin Klein underwear obediently holds out her arms while Lea uses a big wooden spoon to slather them thickly with wax; a minute later, she uses both her thumbs to peel the wax away from each arm in one long sheet. Lea coats the fronts of my legs—from my knees to my ankles—and then turns to Joan's stretcher. We talk about wax while this woman holds her underwear aside and Lea wipes the big spoon across her bikini line. "It hurts less and less each time," Joan tells me. "And the hair grows back lighter and softer."

"And the hair grows back lighter and softer." This is the depilator's credo, an exclusionary logic that elevates one depilatory practice over another, usually with the help of convincing scientific facts. The waxer's logic goes like this: the heat of the wax opens follicles, so the hair is less likely to break off as it is tugged from the follicle. And most important, something in the process changes the follicle, so the hair, when it does return, is softer, lighter, and less offensive than it was originally. This talk is so seductive, the heat and stretch of the wax so reassuring, that I don't prepare for what happens next. Lea reaches under the hardened wax and lifts, swiftly and surely.

"*Ow!*" I yell it, loudly. And again, when she does the other leg. "*Ow!*" I'm surprised, and more than a bit hurt. I've been betrayed by my new friends, and tears spring to my eyes.

Joan is sympathetic. "It always hurts the first time," she offers. "It gets better." But Polish-born Lea isn't taking her cue; my life can't be that hard. "The hair is stronk, because you've been shavink," she says accusingly. This is the flip side of the depilator's credo: following other methods of hair removal always makes hair darker, coarser, and more persistent. "From shavink, the roots get stronk. But why are you screamink?" she asks, clicking her tongue, shaking her head in disbelief, as if she is the one who has been betrayed. "Nobody else is screamink."

Despite the air conditioning, I'm starting to sweat. I think it's because of the pain. Perhaps my nerves can't take this, I reason, and I begin to consider how I might leave gracefully, the backs of my legs still hairy—until I realize that the room is, indeed, getting hotter and hotter. A pot of paraffin, also cooked on Lea's stove next door, has caught fire. Calmly, women in white coats and bobby socks open and shut the door to the little room. I see flames—red and purple—through the doorway, but I've learned, at least, not to scream, so I bite my tongue. I sense that these women feel that beautiful skin is something they know more about than American women (we are, after all, women who shave without realizing the consequences; women who imagine that beauty can be pain-free) and there's something in the way they move with their shoulders instead of their hips that makes me inclined to agree. Suddenly, I'm ashamed to belong to so unenlightened, so feeble, a group. While Lea finishes my legs, I watch these women pour pitchers of water over piles of white sheets, and go in, one by one, to smother the fire.

Persian Wax, $15 Jar

Samantha Bennahum's boyfriend just started shaving his legs—well, actually, he uses Nair—and she thinks it's sweet. The hair was blocking the sun, she explains, and even though he's not a vain person, really, he wanted an even tan. "And," she adds, drawing it out as her voice lowers into a giggle, "he said he wanted to have his smooth legs on my smooth legs."

At twenty-seven Samantha thinks she is finally comfortable with her body hair—but it took a long time to get there. "I'm a pretty hairy person," she says. "Not to the point where I have so much on my back or anything, but . . . I started waxing my legs when I was thirteen. I went through puberty when I was ten." She remembers standing in her grandmother's bathtub, before she learned to shave, trying not to rinse off the bleach that was eating at her face and legs. "It itched; it hurt." She winces even now. "I hated the bleach."

But it wasn't until she was in her midteens that she started to get serious about the hair that was bothering her. "When I was sixteen, I started waxing furiously. I did the toe-to-waist thing. My hair must've been so long . . . it hurt so much." Facial hair, though, was a little more difficult. "I had huge five o'clock shadows. I hated it. I was always teased for it, kids called me 'monkey.'" Shaving her face wasn't an option, since stubble is too "pokey," so she started going to Lucy Peters for electrolysis when she was home on vacation from boarding school. "They had a bar in the changing room—that was how painful it was," she remembers. Too young to drink, Samantha would go to the dentist for Novacain shots before going for electrolysis. But midtown traffic was always a problem, and the Novacain would often wear off before she started her treatment. "I spent fifty hours there and I still have hair on my face," she says with a sigh.

Unwilling to spend fifty dollars or more a month for waxing, she now does it herself, at her apartment in Brooklyn. When it's too hot, and her body sweat makes it impossible for the wax to stick, she goes to her parents' apartment on the Upper East Side of Manhattan—they have air conditioning. A jar of Persian Wax from the Vitamin Shoppe costs her fifteen dollars and lasts for three or four waxings. She spreads it on with a kitchen knife and takes it off with a torn-up pillowcase.

Now, pleased to learn that it doesn't grow back too stubbly, Samantha shaves and plucks whatever facial hair irritates her. "I just take care of those creatures," she says, in the voice of a confident exterminator. "Until I felt comfortable with it, I remember other people being uncomfortable."

But still, there are times when she remembers what it was like to be a hairy ten-year-old on the playground. At a picnic, recently, a friend of her boyfriend's spotted a hair growing from her Adam's apple and had to comment. "So, Samantha, you're growing a beard?"

"Ten years ago, I would've gone off crying," she says. Instead, "I think I went home that night and shaved."

And what did Samantha say to him? "Nice manners." But she was thinking, No wonder you're not married.

Electricity: A History

Nearly a century after Benjamin Franklin flew his famous kite, Dr. Charles Michel, a St. Louis opthalmologist, discovered a new use for traveling ions: disabling troublesome hair follicles. Desperate to help a patient suffering from *trichiasis*—a condition in which eyelashes, instead of curving up and away from the eye, curve toward it, endangering the eyeball—Dr. Michel inserted a needle into the offending follicle, sent electric current through it for over a minute, and generated enough sodium hydroxide, or lye, at the tip of the needle to destroy the papilla, the hair's primary source of nourishment. It was 1875, and Dr. Michel had invented electrolysis. Within twenty years, electrolysis had become both a science and a profession, a fundamental piece of an emerging commercial beauty culture that would tolerate very little superfluous hair.

Perhaps it is a credit to the founding fathers of electrology, or perhaps it's a testament to the profundity of the underlying principles, but the truth is that very little has changed since Dr. Michel's first experiments. In 1891, Nikola Tesla, inventor of the Tesla coil, developed a slightly different technique, using a high frequency current that worked with heat, rather than the chemical reaction of the direct, or galvanic, current. Instead of engendering a chemical exchange between the skin's own water and sodium chloride, producing sodium hydroxide, Tesla's technique used a quick dash of heat to dry up and cauterize the follicle. Diathermy, or electrocoagulation, proved much faster than Dr. Michel's galvanic method, which eventually accommodated six to ten needles at a time, but could still only treat about one hundred hairs in an hour. Tesla's method made it possible to treat hundreds of hairs an hour. Since then, electrology innovations have been of the mix-and-match variety: There is the blend, a technique that combines galvanic and high frequency currents, using heat to speed the action of the sodium hydroxide. Then there are insulated needles that help concentrate the current at the papilla so a higher frequency can be used without burning the skin. Computers can even print records and automatically determine amperage and pulses per second, according to the thickness and depth of the hair. But Dr. Michel's original principles still hold: sent through a needle, straight to the papilla, electricity can destroy hair follicles and remove hair permanently.

This might account for the gravity of the electrology rap, an officiousness that sets it apart from other depilatory methods. Developed at the same time as a burgeoning class of beauty practitioners, trained estheticians who plied their craft in a professional setting, electrology allies itself with a scientific, medicalized approach to superfluous hair. Waxing, shaving, Nair—these are all impermanent solutions; they work quickly, applied with flimsy, disposable accoutrements often by amateur users. Electrologists must train—120 hours in New York, as many as six hundred hours in other states—to use computerized electrical equipment that can alter body tissue permanently.

Hair removal offers a nod to history and necessity, the parents of invention: there was no bikini wax before the bikini, no commercial market for depilatories before flapper dresses exposed legs and armpits, and no electrology until someone decided there was an overgrowth to zap. Michel, Tesla, and others perfected their technique against a backdrop of social biology, an emerging discourse of racial science that defined groups hierarchically, according to physical characteristics and capabilities. The terms we use today to denote cultural status and distance—highbrow/lowbrow—actually have real biological markers rooted in the nineteenth-century fascination with phrenology, the study of skull shapes and proportions. Less sophisticated racial groups were thought to be identifiable by the short, sloping nature of the brow—a low hairline, essentially, bordered by bushy brows. More advanced peoples were thought to have higher, more capacious brows, a signal of their superior brain power. Designated anthropological categories like "Lowbrowed Ape," "Bushman," and, at the top of the scale, "Caucasian," made a connection between hair growth—especially facial hair growth—and cultural sophistication. Developed to combat abnormal, or troublesome, facial hair, electrology quickly became a tool of social uplift.

Electrology was thus an instrument of improvement to be used by those who found themselves on the underside of increasingly rigid social and racial hierarchies. As millions of hirsute immigrants from Southern and Eastern Europe poured into America, America's beauty professionals were able to offer a wide array of services to speed the assimilation process for immigrant women: they could cover beauty marks, shape nails, style hair, and remove lip fuzz safely and permanently.

In his popular book on beauty culture published in 1911, a dermatologist named William Woodbury dubbed hypertrichosis—an overgrowth of hair—"one of the most annoying and humiliating blemishes that can befall the fair face of woman," but he also acknowledged that this judgment might not apply in all cultures. Hair on the female face "lends a disagreeable look of masculinity," he wrote, everywhere "but in Southern Europe." Not surprisingly, it was a "Jewess" whom Woodbury credits with having the "most extraordinary growth on record," a "stout beard of 1,000 hairs." And although Southern Europeans and Jews are the ethnic groups whom Woodbury associates most directly with facial hair problems, he believes there are other sorts of women who are especially prone to abnormal hair growth: unmarried women over thirty, many of whom are schoolteachers; childless women; menopausal women. . . . Indeed, Woodbury admits, facial hair may appear on any woman during puberty, but there is happy news for the afflicted: it may disappear of its own accord, "especially if the girl marries early." If not, there's always electrolysis.

Gillette Good News, $3.99

Lynda Frank and her friend Cathy are walking down Hudson Street in Greenwich Village. It is just after midnight on a Friday evening, and Lynda and Cathy are dressed for a different venue. They've been to the theater and to dinner and are wearing slim skirts and high heels, so we have to walk slowly on the uneven sidewalks. The western border of the Village, Hudson has the feel of a promenade anyway—it's a balmy presummer night and people are loving each other up and down the block, kissing and hugging across the low iron partitions that mark off the sidewalk seating of bars and restaurants. This is the city, of course, diverse and unpredictable, but it's also a visibly gay neighborhood, and Cathy and Lynda feel at home here—they've just left Rubyfruit, a lesbian bar where a picture of Lynda with her two-year-old grandson smiles at you from the foot of the stairs in the entryway. They've been drinking club soda and ginger ale and enjoying each other's company—Cathy is visiting from Atlanta, and though she comes often enough to share the rent for Lynda's midtown apartment, it still seems a rare enough treat to make them stroll leisurely to stretch the evening out.

But as Cathy and Lynda cross Christopher Street, the main artery of the gay West Village, the street made famous by the legendary Stonewall uprising in 1969, two young men bump their bikes up over the curb. They're too young, and their jeans are too baggy, to mark them as part of the crowds that are spilling out of the restaurants and bars along Hudson Street, and when they see Lynda and Cathy they brake abruptly. One of them howls and wings his back wheel to the left. "Hey—you see that?" He roars to his friend: "Tootsie!"

Lynda and Cathy keep walking, backs straight, heads a little lower than before. Out of the side of her mouth, Cathy asks Lynda, "Did you hear that?"

"Yeah," Lynda answers, sighing. "I heard it—'Tootsie.' "

A disappointing but not unpredictable end to a special evening. What Lynda wants, more than anything, is to pass—for men to hold doors open and for waiters to pull out her chair—"to walk down the street and have no one notice me . . ." But she suspects it is the one achievement just beyond her reach. It's much easier, she thinks, for a woman to pass as a man than it is for a man to pass as a woman. "It's okay to be a little guy," she says wistfully, "but big women get looked at." Women can drop their voices, take hormones that will help them grow facial hair, and wear large clothes to cover their figures; men can grow breasts and cover their beards, but they can't grow hips or raise the pitch of their voices easily, and they can't change the size of their frames. People ignore small, effeminate men, says Lynda, but they stop short when they see big-boned men dressed in women's clothes. Sometimes, they call out the first thing that comes to mind—"Tootsie." Much to their chagrin, Lynda and Cathy have failed to pass; they've been "read."

Male cross-dressers like Cathy and Lynda—men who live much of their lives as men, are often married and heterosexual, but who like, even need, to dress and behave as women—get used to margins, boundaries, and borders, the shadowy spaces between realms and roles where meaning, satisfaction, and fulfillment sometimes hide. For Cathy and Lynda, cross-dressing doesn't just mean maintaining two wardrobes, or two names; it means constructing two lives, in two cities. Cathy lives as a man with her wife in Atlanta, and Lynda lives as a man named Len with her wife in northern New Jersey; they both use Lynda's apartment in the theater district as a launch pad for their separate "femme" lives. Full integration is, by nature, impossible (there would be nothing to "cross" if there were no barriers; taboo can be both inhibiting and essential), and what Cathy and Lynda have learned about geography, they have also learned about identity. Lynda and Len inhabit the same body but different worlds; they accompany each other everywhere, but they wear different clothes and have different acquaintances. (I've spent hours talking to Lynda, but I would never know Len if I passed him in the street.) And when I speak to either of them about the other, the neat divisions of our language ossify unhelpfully: Len becomes a guy that Lynda knows intimately; Lynda becomes a gal that Len openly admires. Only sporadically is she "I," and never are they "we."

A cross-dressing friend of Lynda's, Virginia Prince, once assured her that this habit—this necessity—would not turn her life completely upside down, that everything Len and his wife, Marilyn, have built would not get lost in its wake. "It'll go as far as you want it to go," she said. "It's not like heroin." Lynda remembers this when things get confusing, or when it seems like she's pushing the envelope and Marilyn is pushing it back unopened. It reassures her to think that she can hold on to some control, since so much of this life is about martialing and gratifying ornery and contradictory desires. Like many cross-dressers, she convinced herself that this impulse would die down over time, or go away after she was married to a woman she loved. She thought maybe she could just wear women's underwear, occasionally, under her regular clothes, and that would satisfy her. "Guess what?" she asks. "It doesn't go away." The light glints off her glasses as she shakes her head. And wearing underwear under a suit or jeans? "That only worked 'til I was fifty."

One Sunday afternoon, after driving her wife to a baby shower in Brooklyn, Lynda drove herself to a rundown section of Coney Island to visit a doctor she'd heard about who worked with transsexuals. Dressed as Len—a big guy—she pushed past the receptionist and found the doctor at his desk in a back office. "I don't know what I am," she said, eager to get it all out before he turned her away, "but I have these feelings." The doctor nodded, and told her to go into the other room, get undressed, and come back in naked. Lynda did as she was told and walked back into the doctor's office without any clothes. "Okay, get dressed," the doctor told her, after a brief glance up and down. "You're a transvestite [a cross-dresser], not a transsexual [someone who suffers from profound feelings that they have been born into a body of the wrong gender]." He reached this conclusion because Lynda had not covered her penis when she entered the room; she was obviously, he reasoned, not deeply upset with and disgusted by her own genitals, and was therefore not a transsexual. Lynda was bewildered, even a little doubtful, but relieved. After years of struggle, Marilyn's final word had been this: "I can live with a transvestite, but I can't live with a transsexual."

Over the seventeen years that she's been doing this, Lynda has acquired between six and eight wigs, most of which she keeps on cross stands in her apartment because they let the wigs breathe better than those styrofoam heads. Her favorite is an expensive short blond wig—three hundred dollars—that she bought on Fifty-seventh Street at a wig salon where she could try wigs on at a private booth in the back. Before buying that wig, she had tried to buy wigs that matched her dark eyebrows, but then she started to notice that a lot of old ladies wear blond wigs. Lynda's conclusion: "They make you look a lot younger." A young woman who worked at the wig salon helped her choose the cut and shade, letting Lynda feel that her shopping there, at a women's wig salon, was a perfectly natural choice.

Lynda's wig regimen requires time, energy, and money—all of which she is willing to invest, because these wigs are an essential part of her persona. She's just purchased a styling head and table clamps from a beauty supply shop around the corner from her apartment, and she's planning to work on washing and styling her wigs herself, since she hasn't found a place where she's entirely comfortable dropping them off. Years ago, she experimented with wig cement to hold her wig in place, but lately she's been using a wig cap. Made of a stretchy rubber, the wig cap molds to Lynda's head and, along with the "wig catcher" clips she uses in each side and at the back of her head, holds her wig in place. It's clear, as we discuss the details of her routine, that Lynda has enjoyed forging beauty rituals for herself, discarding wig cement in favor of the wig cap, deciding that clips hold better than bobby pins. Wigs are part of a beauty system that she guards carefully, even ferally, because they contain the essence of her femininity, a quality that for many years she had no means to express. When I comment on her nails she looks surprised, and maybe a little bit hurt. "I *polished* them," she says, "you call it *paint*?"

Ultimately, though, Lynda would like to be able to wear her own hair and do away with the wigs entirely. She points to the wig she is wearing, a short wavy bouffant that frames her face and just brushes the back of her neck.

"This would be my ideal hairstyle—wavy, not too curly, and *feminine*." Considering this possibility, I ask what Len's hair is like and she smiles mischievously. "Len's hair has *changed*!" She waves away my wonder with her hand. "Len has a ponytail!" Hoping one day to be able to style her own hair into Lynda's coif, she's been cultivating what grows beneath the wig. "It's nice to be glamorous," she says, acknowledging that what she's attempting might not exactly be the hippest, hottest style, "but for me, it's most important to look feminine, to pass. I don't mind looking like someone's old aunt."

Body hair poses a different set of problems for Lynda and Len. For months now, Len has been growing head hair that will, with any luck, prove useful to Lynda. Len's body hair, however, is something Lynda doesn't need. Beards first. Shaving with an electric razor, as has always been Len's custom—*not* as close as a blade, says Lynda emphatically—gets Lynda through the night, along with Beard Cover, an orangy makeup designed to counteract the bluish cast of five o'clock shadow, and Cover Girl beige foundation. (No powder—it cakes, then flakes.) Bodies second. "I have a good time with body hair," says Lynda, laughing a little self-consciously, "I shave it off." An hour in the shower, once a week, with shaving cream and a Gillette safety razor, and her skin is smooth and clean. Feminine. "Little Len liked the hair," says Lynda, referring to her younger self and a time when she was proud of body hair and the implied masculinity. "Big Len likes it shaved." Marilyn can stand anything, it seems, except stubble. "Then she kicks me out of bed." Lynda's once-a-week body shave seems to suit them both.

Like the wave and curl of Lynda's wigs, a hairless body is an important part of her fashion understatement, her desire to become, on the surface at least, an ordinary, invisible woman. Lynda enjoys sleeveless shirts, nude stockings, and strapless gowns, and dark body hair, in her estimation, goes with none of these. For occasions like the Rubyfruit Sweetheart Ball, where Lynda has worn her custom-made strapless gowns—"Oooh! They'll knock your socks off!"—Marilyn was an obliging date and shaved her back, which, normally, Lynda can't reach and leaves alone. But as with the bedtime stubble, Marilyn has lines she just can't cross: she can accept a hairless Len with a lengthening ponytail, but a Len with tweezed eyebrows is going too far. "Marilyn will get mad if it's too extreme," says Lynda, a bit glum when we discuss the dramatic possibilities of eyebrow shaping.

Tellingly, Lynda too seems a bit nervous when it seems Len's male grooming is being left behind. "I like the masculine role, and I like the feminine role." She outlines her dilemma carefully, noting both her growing attachment to Lynda's life and her need to maintain Len's. "I probably like the feminine role a teensy, weensy bit better." If everything else was equal, she would probably dress as Lynda most mornings. Wistfully, Lynda imagines life as a lesbian. "I thought that'd be fun," she says, as if it is a profession she was steered away from. But everything else is not equal: Len owned a gas station in his town, is a past president of his synagogue, has a wife, children, and grandchildren he loves. Lynda goes back to the diagnosis of the Coney Island doctor and remembers she is a cross-dresser, not a transsexual.

The problem, now, comes down to fashion and boundaries: how to bolster two lives, two wardrobes, two body images, two hairstyles. Len crosses the street whenever he can, dodging traffic with a jog; Lynda waits for the light. "Lynda can't run," she says. "Not in this skirt." Len used to be a snappy dresser, but now it's Lynda's turn. "Don't get me wrong—Len doesn't look like a *schlunk*, but he doesn't take the care that Lynda does." And Len is having trouble with his old friends and relationships; he's getting impatient with straight men lately. Men want to convey information, prove things, Lynda says, following the wisdom of John Gray and Deborah Tannen, but "women talk to get closer to people." She pauses. "I think Lynda wants to get closer to people." As she says this, her bare arm brushes against mine and I feel stubble. At first it prickles, and then, on second thought, it doesn't at all.

Electricity, $100/hour

Most electrologists are former clients, and as such, they carry within them both the fervor of the convert and the gratitude of the supplicant. A registered nurse and an electrologist for twenty years, Myriam Vasicka also channels the wisdom of a social scientist and the compassion of a psychotherapist. "People come when they have so many things unresolved." She shakes her head for emphasis and her black bob swings against her cheek. "Any emotional stress, there will be hair growth. It's like a clock—if one thing's off, everything's off." For many of Myriam's clients, conquering unwanted hair is the first step toward mastering other difficulties. "People think, if I can change this, maybe I can stop smoking!" For those who've obsessed long and hard about their problem, electrology might provide a much-needed respite. "When they give up, it's better." Myriam's voice is calm and reassuring; her office is a soothing cream-colored cubicle lodged in the bottom of a doorman building on upper Park Avenue. They can tell themselves, "This is Myriam's problem now."

Years of experience have allowed Myriam to rank hair according to its susceptibility to her electrically charged needle. Red and blond hairs are the hardest to treat, she says, since they are often nearly invisible and deceptively strong. The coarse, dark, curly hair of Central Europeans—Greeks and Jews—is also tough, deeply rooted, and intransigent. But many of Myriam's customers are Jewish, and Myriam finds that their determined approach to hair removal compensates for the depth of their follicles. "Jewish people change things; they have the means or they find the means. And . . ." She pauses for a second, not sure if she'll offend. "Well, Jewish women are very vain. They do it the way it's supposed to be done." Myriam admires this. Despite her tall girl's slouch, she is also something of a drill instructor, and she makes sure that I understand that electrology is not a truly quick fix. "Coming here requires discipline and commitment," she says sternly, her Uruguayan accent crossing her *t*s. "If people don't come regularly, then the process won't work."

Hair that has been repeatedly waxed and tweezed is also problematic for Myriam's needle—deeper, darker, and more stubborn than it might otherwise have been. "It gets worse and worse, coarser and curlier," says Myriam, frustrated by the claims of waxing salons that promise hair will return finer and finer until it disappears altogether. The real result, says Myriam, is ingrown hairs that take even longer to destroy with electrolysis, since it must first straighten the follicle in order for the needle to reach the papilla. "What they say is not accurate."

Myriam is equally skeptical when it comes to the sometimes extravagant claims of centers offering the latest laser technology. Not wanting to be left behind, when the new technology came on the market she trained with a doctor and worked on people with lasers, and frankly, she's not impressed. Much like electrolysis, lasers work by damaging the blood vessels that nourish the hair and allow it to grow, but Myriam's noticed that those damaged blood vessels seem to heal themselves and go back to work in eight weeks. At best, she says, lasers are a temporary method of hair removal. "It lasts longer than waxing," she offers. "No one will tell you its permanent." (Indeed, lasers have only been FDA-approved for hair "reduction," not "removal.") Many of her clients are eager to try lasers, especially on large areas for which electrolysis is too costly and time consuming, like a woman's legs or a man's back, and Myriam considered expanding her office to accommodate the larger machines. But she just can't bring herself to recommend it. "You have to believe, whatever you do. I don't knock any of it," she says, referring to the whole gamut of hair removal options. She's almost ready to apologize for her own success, but then thinks better of it, since the truth is actually very simple. "Electrolysis is the only one that works."

Myriam's clients react to her combination of hearty discipline and maternal omnipotence exactly as you'd expect:

some submit, with a sigh of relief; others act out. Rachel, a twenty-six-year-old magazine editor with the pale skin and fine, dark hair that make her an ideal candidate for Myriam's needle, kicks subtly at Myriam's regime, sometimes arriving "two or three" minutes late for her biweekly appointments. Always contrite, she complains of subway delays, but both she and Myriam know the truth: it's Rachel that's late, not the train.

Though she is completely dedicated to Myriam, Rachel concedes that she's had a long history of ambivalence about electrology and the circumstances that have led her to spend nearly three thousand dollars, so far, on her bikini line. When she was a sophomore in high school, she used the backdoor of a beauty salon to visit her mother's electrologist. "I hated it," she says. "It was before Emla [an anaesthetic cream]. It was endless . . . it was boring." She stops short but it seems the list goes on. The electrologist hurt her, and listened to loud talk radio; she was too chatty, and too friendly with Rachel's mother. Extremely self-conscious, the teen-aged Rachel told none of her friends about her visits to the electrologist, and not wanting anyone—acquaintance or stranger—to see her with a telltale white mustache, she hid her face on the car ride over to the salon when the numbing benefits of Emla finally became available. Trying to make her feel better, the electrologist passed on the name of a popular schoolmate who was also submitting to the prick of the electric needle, but her violation did little to set Rachel at ease. Rachel adopts Myriam's stern tone when she speaks of this woman, so clearly Myriam's professional opposite. "That wasn't very discreet of her, was it?"

These memories of high school hair trouble seem vivid

today, a string of worries that lead back along familiar, bumpy paths. Rachel's wedding, which she and her mother have been planning for months, will be held in her parents' backyard next week, and the intricate knots of family ties are standing in high relief. Recently, her mother visited for an intense week of mother-daughter bonding complete with fittings, fights, and finally, a bridal shower. About to cross the proverbial threshold, it's time for Rachel to take her life and her story in hand, but parts of it are slippery, hard to grasp. In high school, fashion demanded that excess hair be eradicated swiftly, silently, and completely. Rachel remembers the urgency and now tries her best to explain. She is articulate, of course, and speaks with an editor's precise grammar, but adolescent angst sometimes defies reason. "We wore short uniforms!" she cries. And then, "I was one of six Jewish girls in my class . . . I was pretty comfortable with myself, but that was something I was grossed out by."

I'm interested in the association: in Los Angeles, where Rachel grew up, was hairiness a Jewish problem? She stops short, not sure if that sounds exactly right. There's a connection all right, but it might not simply be a matter of ethnic association. "I don't know if it's that," she says finally, "or if it's just—my dad." Family is always more complicated than sociology. She hesitates, but then decides that after all, so near her wedding, a new life and "victory" over her unwanted hair, it's worth a laugh. "I come from a family of very furry people. It's soft and fine and dark and a *lot*. We call my father 'Bear Man.' "

Truly, though, it's her mother whom Rachel's been tangling with all these years. "She doesn't shave her armpits, but she's completely hair phobic." Rachel looks around the crowded café near her office where we are eating lunch. She is trying to explain, or decide, how a supportive, empathic mother, a careful psychotherapist who doesn't believe in makeup and has always counseled self-love, can also be behind her ambivalence about herself, her decisions, and her body hair. During her freshman year of college, Rachel stopped shaving her legs, but continued to visit her mother's chatty electrologist on vacations, slipping in the backdoor, an Emla mustache behind her hand. She also stopped eating, a silent protest against appetite and imposition. "I was at war with my body," she says now.

Resenting her mother's input, she hadn't yet discovered the boundaries where maternal demand ended and personal necessity began. Everyone around her at college seemed earthy and natural, but also smooth-skinned and athletic; she felt bookish and hairy. On a family trip to Yosemite, her brother looked at her unshaven legs and pronounced them "disgusting." She wasn't sure if she agreed or not. By the end of her sophomore year, she was shaving and eating again, but the old tug-of-war wasn't over.

When Rachel's mother visited this past month, she asked Rachel to set up an appointment with Myriam. She didn't say what she wanted treated, and Rachel didn't ask. As the day neared, Rachel got more and more nervous, sure her mother would find fault with the person she trusted—the professional aide she'd found completely on her own. Somehow, she felt sure the meeting of these two important women would be used against her. "Your mother's seeing some very personal part of your life that she's not usually privy to," she says. "I knew something had to go wrong." Of course it did: a scheduling glitch forced the usually punctual and exacting Myriam to cancel Rachel's mother's appointment. Myriam was "hugely apologetic," and her mother didn't seem angry, but Rachel provoked an argument anyway. Remembering, she balls her fists like a two-year-old and scowls at the ghost of her mother that hovers nearby. "Of course you didn't like her," she pouts, "because she's *mine*."

Now she laughs—even her fiancé told her she was being ridiculous. She might even be relieved, in the end, that her mother didn't lean back in that chair that's so familiar to her and chat with the person Rachel admits is both beauty consultant and confidant. Her parents pay for her treatment, and she's "gotten past" feeling badly about asking for money as an adult. "That," she says, "is the advantage of having a furry family." They pay money to undo the havoc wrought by their own genes. But she's knows what she's going to do when her work with Myriam is finished and she has a spare hour in her increasingly busy schedule. She raises the dark, dramatic eyebrows Myriam has helped her shape, and smiles. "I'm going for therapy," she says. "I'm going to work out those issues about my mom."

Light, $1200, Chin

Dara, who is petite, pretty, and remarkably hairless, does not shave her upper thighs. The hair there is very light and bothers her very little, and she doesn't want "to do anything to mess it up." Her job is to introduce prospective customers, who arrive daily at this Manhattan laser center for the free consultations advertised all over the city, to the depilatory prowess of the Softlight laser. While she takes down information about my health, medications, and hair growth, she is sharing some of her own experiences and observations. She does her bikini once with the laser, and she's "good for the whole summer." To Dara, this is worth the $360 one treatment costs because it is a step toward permanence—probably—and also because it allows more freedom than waxing, another preferred method of bikini depilation. "I can put on a bathing suit whenever I want!" Dara is still impressed by this facet of the laser operation— longevity is important in the summer.

Dara inquires about my depilatory history and clucks her tongue in disapproval, though not in despair. "Plucking, of course, you know, is *the* worst thing you can do," she says sorrowfully. "It stimulates growth." She hears the same sad, misguided story over and over again: "Clients come in and say, 'I had one or two hairs and then—'" Dara claps her hand to the bottom of her chin. "Boom!" Oops—a beard. "It's *because* they plucked!"

With the arrival of laser technology, the world of depilation is starting to resemble a Hollywood action movie: there are the enemies—the hairs—advancing in a dark, dangerous formation over hilly, innocent territory; there are the victims, earnest, well-meaning Americans who merely want to be free and safe; and there are the heroes, hardworking scientists pushed to deploy sophisticated instruments they don't fully understand because the fate of the world is at stake. Sunny, smart, and eternally hopeful, laser technicians and doctors alike refer to their lasers respectfully, cautiously, and anthropomorphically, as if they can't quite believe that they're for real, but maybe they are and maybe they're human. And, indeed, these laser have names that reinforce their surreality. They are names that evoke historical mightiness—Alexandrite—and names that foretell technological sophistication beyond the layperson's puny imagination—ND/YAG, and Coherent Lightseer Diode. "I think lasers are a whole new world!" one doctor quipped jubilantly.

Originally used by dermatologists for skin resurfacing and scar and tattoo removal, lasers have recently become dermatology's secret weapon against unwanted hair. They even work like weapons, using simple scientific principles—some substances absorb some wavelengths more than others—to target and destroy enemy strongholds. The laser emits light at a wavelength that will, hopefully, be well absorbed by the melanin, or pigment, in the interior of the hair follicle; the energy of that light will then work like the heat of an electrolysis needle, coagulating the blood vessels in the follicle. One doctor, quoted in the *New York Times*, likened lasers to "smart bombs." Dr. Kenneth Rothaus, an Upper East Side plastic surgeon, explains the action of his YAG laser as a "surge" of energy that "disrupts the entire hair shaft," finally causing the melanin to "explode."

Right now, doctors and scientists are trying to understand which wavelengths will penetrate deepest and work for the most ranges of melanin, since some lasers, like the Ruby, seem to have limited effect on lighter hair—i.e., hair with less melanin. Others, like Softlight, are used with a carbon gel that is supposed to penetrate the hair shaft, thus providing pigmentation where it may be lacking. At the same time, the cumulative energy of the procedure has to be taken into consideration. If too little heat is generated, the hair shaft will live on—injured, perhaps, but not disabled—but a high peak energy sent into the skin for too long a time will burn it. Though it is too soon to tell unequivocally, Dr. Rothaus thinks that his Alexandrite laser, which has a wavelength of 755 nanometers and fires for five to ten seconds at a time, will probably prove more effective at actually eliminating hair. On the other hand, the Alexandrite is often uncomfortable for patients, especially those doing sensitive areas like the upper lip. For these patients, Dr. Rothaus might recommend the YAG, which uses a wavelength of 1064 nanometers, the same as the Softlight, but quickly administered, with a high peak energy that penetrates deeply but doesn't generate as much surface heat and is therefore easier to endure than the Alexandrite. This laser, Dr. Rothaus knows, sends follicles into a prolonged telogen—rest phase—but he suspects that fewer of them will remain in telogen than with the Alexandrite. "It scares them," he says, but it might not kill them. Still, the YAG is clearly his favorite new toy. Small, sleek, and relatively unobtrusive, about the size of a small robot with a plastic arm on top, the YAG may become the new rich girl's wax. Its effects will last longer, and, over time, it will probably accomplish what so many waxes promise: lighter, finer hair that eventually disappears.

Although the FDA has set up clear distinctions between "removal" and "reduction," making it illegal for laser practitioners to promise to remove hair permanently, laser territory has a boomtown feel to it. It is a giddy, wild frontier that the combination of hope and technology have placed just beyond the serious reach of the law. So far, anyone who can pay the price of a machine—anywhere from $40,000–$250,000—and receive a training certificate can use it. And the semantic difference between reduction and removal, perhaps an obvious one on the pages of *Webster's Collegiate*, is often buried beneath a mountain of bareskin ads and the well-meaning promises of converted technicians.

Vanishing Point, a laser hair removal chain that began in Florida and has sprouted like a crop of new-grown hair across the country, has New York offices just off Union Square in a sleek, smooth blond-wood space adorned with color photos of hairless torsos, legs, pubes, and faces. Their magic bullet is the Epilight, a machine that is not, technically, a laser but works a lot like one. The Epilight is a pulse light that uses a larger spectrum of wavelengths than a laser, thus making it effective, theoretically, for a wider variety of skin and hair types. Equipped with a computer that filters out unnecessary or ineffective wavelengths, the Epilight is celebrated as smarter, less painful, less expensive, and less time-consuming than electrolysis and other light epilatories. It is, according to Vanishing Point's carefully schooled staff, "as close to permanent as you can get."

Robin, my Vanishing Point technician, tells me that along with former waxers, tweezers, and electrolysis clients, she sees a lot of disappointed laser users as well. In part, she admits, this might be a matter of finances: a package of four half-hour visits costs $750 at Vanishing Point, whereas it could cost as much as $1,500 at a doctor's office. But she believes it is also Vanishing Point's superior technology that accounts for its popularity. Open only seven months, they are booking for October when I visit in July, and planning the opening of another salon on the Upper West Side. A former electrologist, Robin is an emphatic convert, warning that waxing and plucking actually stimulate the lymphatic system, causing more hair to grow than ever before. She repeats Vanishing Point's carefully boastful refrain—"It's as close to permanent as you can get"—adding, with a smile, "and it doesn't hurt!"

Helen, a thirty-one-year-old former waxer, flinches behind her protective dark glasses when Robin zaps her bikini area with the laser, but, on a scale of one to ten, Helen rates the Epilight a one and waxing a twenty.

My own experience is uneventful, but also inconclusive. Having decided that it is best to treat a whole area, and that I was more willing to expose my armpits than my bikini area to a stranger wielding hot light, I allowed Robin to zap my stubbly underarms one summer afternoon. After discreetly asking my "heritage" (East European Jews get a II on the Epilight computer; Hispanic people get a V), Robin set the machine and spread on a cool, clear gel that resembles ultrasound jelly on my armpit. I put on my protective glasses, while she assured me that she closes her eyes when the light flashes and doesn't need glasses for herself, and then . . . zap! Immediately, I smelled that acrid odor of burning hair, and sure enough, when Robin scraped off the gel with a tongue depressor, some of the eighth of an inch of stubble necessary for treatment went along with it, having just been torched right out of the follicle. A week later, as predicted, most of the rest of the hair fell out, and what didn't simply stopped growing. After another week, I got sick of watching the few lingering hairs and finally shaved.

Not being a scientist, I will admit that I ruined the control, and a month later exposed my underarms to Dr. Rothaus's beloved YAG, which turned whatever brave hairs I had left a sad, defeated white. Some of them fell out on their own. But no miracle has occurred; there is still life left in my follicles. This is all I know for sure: true to Dr. Rothaus's contention, the YAG is much less painful than either the Epilight or the Alexandrite. Now two months since the first light zap, I have far less hair growing under my arms than I did before, and in the shower, when I don't need to shave, I've been feeling an incipient panic: what if I want it back?

Electricity, $45/hour

Myriam Vasicka once had a client who was born a man, but considered herself a woman. Estrogen supplements made this girl's skin gorgeous—"peaches and cream," swears Myriam—but it only lightened her body hair; much of it, including her beard, had to be treated with electrolysis. Three or four times a week, this girl sat in Myriam's chair for hour-long sessions; one year and $20,000 later, her beard was nearly gone, though maintenance, Myriam estimates, cost her nearly $400 a month for another three or four years. "Hair is so important to them." Myriam says this sadly, knowing that for her transgendered and transsexual clients, having too much hair growing in the wrong places can be a significant barrier to the creation of a new identity. And yet, their very presence in her chair signals that something has gone awry; electrolysis is only a small part of the solution. "Nature teases this person, and she's not a man." Myriam leans forward and lowers her voice. She's trying to master the story, to explain how one goes from being a man to being a woman—or doesn't really. "I have to call her 'her,' but she's a he." Myriam is compassionate, and is willing to experiment with pronouns, but like most people, she believes in the bottom line.

We modern Westerners are a people dedicated to the bottom line. In a world of shifting markets and fast-moving commodities, the bottom line is what keeps us safe and grounded. Simply put, we expect sex—essentially, a set of biological factors—and gender—the culturally acknowledged expression of maleness and femaleness, or masculinity and femininity—to match. Even in places where it appears subversions are on the agenda, we've clung to the ideal of a fixed external reality. Though the origin of the term *drag* is not known, some suspect that it was originally an acronym: *D*ressed *A*s a *G*irl, a construction that has at its center a simile that highlights the norm. Guys dressed *like* girls are not, after all, girls.

Transgender is an umbrella term that gathers beneath it a range of gender-defying individuals, including cross-dressers, the intersexed (hermaphrodites), nonoperative transsexuals (people who live as individuals of the opposite gender without plans for sex-reassignment surgery), and postoperative transsexuals. Vague and amorphous, it is the perfect designation for a group that is not a group; it is, in essence, an antiterm meant to signal a defiance or discomfort with the norm, the perfect coincidence of word and meaning, biology and gender. The *New York Times* reports that over fifteen hundred Americans a year undergo some sort of sex-reassignment surgery, in an effort to rectify what is clinically and somewhat pessimistically called "gender dysphoria," a profound discomfort with the assigned sex and gender of one's birth. Given a psychiatric diagnosis and a plan of treatment, many of us might feel compassion for the transsexual individual, who is, after all, fighting an acknowledged disease. But where acceptance and sympathy can follow, final understanding often stops short. If gender dysphoria and sex reassignment are necessities we can grasp, letting go is still a problem: America's first transsexual, Christine Jorgensen, was never just Christine; she was always Christine-who-used-to-be-George.

In the standards of care outlined by the Harry Benjamin International Gender Dysphoria Association, there are specific steps to be followed along the way to a surgical change of gender. The most significant hurdle is the Real Life Test, a year spent living full-time as a person of the opposite gender. Meant to school a surgical candidate in the skills of living as a new man or woman, it is also an exhausting transition accomplished with counseling, wardrobe changes, hormone shots, electrolysis, and sundry other preparations, but without the benefit of surgical completion. Stefanie Schumacher, who is thirty-six and lives with her parents in Gainesville, Georgia, lost her job as a manager at a 7-Eleven during her Real Life Test. She finished her transition at the more accepting Kmart, where she managed the small appliance and kitchen corner, but she still remembers the feeling of vulnerability that haunted her after her departure from

7-Eleven. "We're a very small minority. We're not protected." At moments like this, Stefanie's voice is insistent, but even over the phone she sounds nervous and scared.

Stefanie's identification with girls "goes back as far as I can remember," even though, as a young Steven, she often must have seemed a typical little boy. She played baseball, had G.I. Joes, and liked girls, but at ten she discovered her mother's clothes. "I remember getting dressed up, lying down, and closing my eyes and wishing I would wake up a girl." At sixteen, she read an article in *Playboy* about the transsexual Wendy Carlos, and suddenly, everything made sense. "I had a pretty normal existence—I looked like a guy and I was attracted to girls." But the Carlos article helped Steven sort out his discomfort with being a boy. "Oh, my God," he said. "That's me." Increasingly confused, Steven finally sought counseling after dropping out of college. "I didn't know anything about anything," Stefanie remembers. "I told the therapist, 'This body's not for me.' "

It took years of denial, two different therapists, a stint with the Hare Krishnas, a fling with alcohol and a Pentecostal church, and increasing suicidal despair to finally bring Stefanie to a diagnosis and an understanding of the problem. When a transgendered woman named Anastasia began to work with her at the 7-Eleven in Gainesville, Stefanie took action. She asked Anastasia for help. "She became my drag mother. She taught me everything." Most important, Anastasia and her friends treated Stefanie as Stefanie, not as a freak, and not as Steven. Later, Stefanie approached another transsexual and asked for help in obtaining estrogen, finally buying black market shots for fifty dollars apiece, four times the prescription cost. By the time Stefanie found the therapist and doctor who presided over her official transition, she was already in transition, growing breasts and losing body hair.

As Steven, Stefanie had found it increasingly difficult to face the mirror. Even after shaving, her beard was thick and heavy, a bristly reminder of a reality she'd rather forget. "I had a little monster between my legs and this shit on my face." Still she's disgusted. Now, a year after she began electrolysis, Stefanie is finally beginning to see the light at the end of the tunnel. But the journey has been unpleasant, frustrating, and painful. "I've cried in the chair," she says, her voice soft and sad. "I think it's never gonna be over." She loves her electrologist, but curses her with each zap on her upper lip. So far, she's done over one hundred hours of electrolysis, twice a week at the beginning and once a week now, as she can afford it. At forty-five dollars an hour, she's spent a little less than half of what she paid for her surgery after taking a second mortgage on her parents' house. (She got a discount for having a rhinoplasty, vaginoplasty, and breast augmentation all at once. The total was $11,600, and that included a two-week stay at a recuperation residence in Canada.) Another ten hours, she thinks, and she'll be clear, though estimates are only that—just estimates. Some of her hairs have been treated fifteen, twenty-five times. "It's an imperfect science." She sighs.

But since her surgery, Stefanie has been feeling hopeful and satisfied. "From the physical standpoint, I'm a woman. I'm complete." She hasn't really tried out her new vagina yet, but she's "extremely pleased" with it nonetheless. With bubbly enthusiasm, she sounds like a true southern belle. "There's nothing left to cut off!" She's beginning to see her weekly visits to the electrologist as akin to the forty milligram shots of del-estrogen she receives every other week as part of her routine feminine maintenance. Electrolysis, she thinks, was a tougher test of her womanly perseverance than surgery. "If you're willing to deal with that needle, you're willing to get your balls cut off."

Pink Polyester Thread, $8, Eyebrows

When I first meet Monica, she is holding a folded tissue dipped in astringent to her upper lip, gingerly daubing at a patch of skin that has turned an angry red. Underneath each of her eyebrows, there is also a telltale line, pink and puffy. She touches the tissue to these, too, and when she stands up to look at her face in the mirror above her chair, she frowns. This is her first visit to Sunita, an esthetician who works at My Place Too, a salon tucked at the bottom of a big midtown Manhattan office complex, where men and women in gray suits run down the escalator to get their nails done during their midmorning coffee break. A documentary filmmaker, Monica doesn't work in this neighborhood; she has traveled to come here, lured by an article that recommended Sunita as an expert *threader*, someone skilled in the Asian art of removing superfluous hair with, yes, thread. Indeed, it's true: Sunita wields her spool of Singer thread like a parade majorette, winding and spinning until the motion itself looks like magic—a bow sliding on violin strings, not thread plucking lip hair.

Sunita herself is nonplussed by Monica's discomfort. She peers quickly under Monica's tissue and pronounces her fine. "A little irritation," she says, shrugging, "is normal."

At the foot of her worktable, Sunita keeps a tiny hot pot of DD wax, spiked with lemon and honey, for customers who want to remove body hair, or for those who are afraid to try threading on their faces. Indeed, more than half of Sunita's clientele are "too chicken" to let her use her snazzy pink thread, even though Sunita insists it is the best way to approach the sensitive and precise art of removing facial hair. Waxing pulls and stretches the skin—that's okay for your legs, says Sunita, but not for your face. To demonstrate, she unwinds about a foot of thread, twists it into an unfinished noose, an oblong loop wound together at the end, and uses a pulley motion—the circumference of the noose twists together and rips out a line of hairs, one by one, along her own puffed out upper lip. It's like plucking, only faster and more efficient. "It's natural—no harm," says Sunita, firmly believing that the pain of pulling hairs from your upper lip does not constitute harm. "But you have to use polyester." She points to her spool of SuperStrong thread. "It's stronger—less elastic than cotton." The pink is just for fun.

By the time I see Monica a week later, her eyebrows and upper lip are again pale and fine. Her skin seems delicate, almost translucent, but nothing in the way she moves suggests that she is. She's tall, lean, and purposeful, her body suspended from ample shoulders. She doesn't remember the beauty politics of Tulsa, Oklahoma, her hometown, being as complicated as they are in the East. "There were two groups at my high school," she recalls. "The ones that shaved and the ones that didn't. I didn't feel strongly enough about leg hair to belong to either group." Monica shaved her legs back then, but she did it "out of boredom" more than anything else. It wasn't until college, when she became acquainted with her boyfriend Jonas's mother, a beauty parlor regular, that she considered removing other body hair. Even then, it was a grudging, gradual process, a slow courtship between Monica and Mrs. Goldberg.

"I never did my nails, or my eyebrows, or anything," says Monica, her cigarette still while her fingers drum the table at an East Village coffee shop near her apartment. "But Jonas's mother gets a manicure every Saturday." Whenever Monica and Jonas visited his parents, in Bethesda, Maryland, Mrs. Goldberg would press Monica to join her. At first, Monica declined, uncomfortable with beauty rituals in general and with Mrs. Goldberg, with whom she felt she had nothing in common. "I thought it was totally self-indulgent. People wax their arms! My mother comes from a poor background, she doesn't go in for this kind of stuff." But Mrs. Goldberg kept pressing her until eventually, after a year and a half of refusals, Monica agreed to accompany her on a Saturday morning beauty jaunt. "That's how we started—it was the manicure," Monica says, as if discussing the early stages of addiction. From there, Monica moved on to a pedicure, and then to a makeup session with Tara, the woman who introduced Monica to threading. That's how she began doing her eyebrows.

At Tara's suggestion, Monica allowed her eyebrows to be waxed, but even now, she remembers her ambivalence. "I didn't have a problem with my eyebrows until she said that," she says. She felt the same when Tara suggested she do her upper lip. "No one ever said, 'Oh, you've got a mustache.' If there were dark hairs there, I hadn't noticed. And it was a nightmare," at first, painful and irritating. Eventually, Tara, who is Indian, started using thread. And even though threading was painful, too—"like mini–razor blades running across your skin"—it was "cleaner than wax and faster than tweezing." Monica seems grateful, and is now unfazed by the pain. "I've been raised with a suck-it-up attitude," she says, inhaling on her cigarette. "It could be the worst pain in the world, and I'd never know it."

Years later, though she and Jonas are not married, Monica thinks she has finally built a familial relationship with Mrs. Goldberg. "I felt her being a little warmer with me. Before, she'd ignore me—she felt as uncomfortable as I did. Now, this is our mother and daughter-in-law thing to do together, something we both understand. Sort of." Monica thinks that Jonas's parents even think it's okay she's not Jewish. Among the Saturday morning beauty parlor crowd—what Monica wryly calls the "yenta scene"—she's finally been promoted. "It's not 'there's Jonas's *friend*,' it's 'there's Jonas's *girlfriend*.' "

Still, Monica has her doubts. It's been four years since she first did her eyebrows, and Jonas is still pushing her to "admit it's kind of fun." She concedes that she likes how it looks, and that it is easier now for her to accept Mrs. Goldberg's attentions. "If she wants to go to Bendel's, and buy something for me, sure, I'll take it. This is the only way she has of communicating," she says. But she's still not sure that this beauty business isn't about vanity and self-indulgence. The threading, the waxing, the brighter blond she's become (Mrs. Goldberg said, "Why don't you get highlights?") seem sometimes like a decadence she's fallen prey to since she came east. With earnest pride and a self-critical eye, Monica compares herself with what she left behind.

Her grandmother, who lives in Elk Horn City, Kentucky, three hours from Lexington on the Virginia border, gets her waist-length hair "done" for five dollars on special occasions. For Monica's sister's graduation in Tulsa, she put it up with butterfly pins. When Monica started working, she sent her grandmother five dollars a month, for a treat, so she could go to the beauty parlor. But Monica suspects that her grandmother isn't spending the money, and she's a little worried her grandmother will think her extravagant. "I don't think she's gone in but once. She's gotten self-conscious. She'll probably give it all back to me when she sees me."

Monica's other grandmother cut her long hair after her husband died. She told Monica she didn't have anyone to look nice for anymore.

No Razors, Wax, or Nair: Free

I'm at a bridal shower and, of course, the talk turns from brides and grooms to grooming and finally, to hair. This is a group where sixties nostalgia lives on and expresses itself in the folds of life—in the toys you buy your kids, the food you cook, and the hair on your body.

Leslie remembers being twelve and finding the first hair in her armpit. In a panic, she called her mother at a bridge game. "She said, 'It's okay, it's normal,' etc., etc. Then, a couple of months later, I find out she'd *told* her bridge group, and they'd had a laugh at my expense." Leslie sits back on the couch and eats some of the shrimp she's brought for this gathering; her son is at home with her husband, her mother's probably playing bridge somewhere in Westchester County, a suburb of New York City, and this business still angers her, more than twenty-five years later. "I was so upset, I didn't shave until I was thirty."

Her mother, like many mothers, believed in "neat," "clean," and hairless. "She gets extremely upset if one pubic hair is peeking out of the bathing suit." Call it rebellion, revenge, or better yet, *reason*—Leslie still won't shave her pubic area. "I don't think it looks bad, and I don't think it's that important!"

Her tale is spinning faster now, fueled by resentment and pride. A leggy California blond she met when her Teen Tour group stopped for refreshment told her it was okay that she didn't shave her legs. " 'I don't shave, and I'm a babe,' she said." Leslie noticed this babe had a hot California guy in tow and decided not to worry about her leg hair, either. Now, she sometimes shaves her legs, but she's spotted a couple of chin hairs, and she doesn't pluck them like she probably should. "I shave them," she says, with a momentary lapse into hair worry shaking her confidence. "That's probably bad. They're probably going to grow back twice as strong, but . . ." She shrugs her "oh well," but still looks relieved when I tell her that's a myth.

Now she remembers a blind date with a fashion photographer. "He studied my face for a long time, and finally said, 'You know, you're really beautiful, but you need to do something about those eyebrows.' So I said, 'Memo to myself: never touch eyebrows.' I don't even own a pair of tweezers."

The bride says that it was her desire to be a hippie that kept her from shaving after that first time she tried it with a rusty disposable she found in the bathroom closet—rebelling against her mother was only a bonus. She shaves her legs now, but can't stand the idea of shaving her armpits—she shudders and clamps her arms at her sides as if it might happen if she didn't stand guard. In fact, she's never shaved her armpits, ever. But it's light hair, she says, reassuring the rest of us who try, in turn, to reassure her. "If I lift my arms at the beach, no one would even notice." Of course they wouldn't.

Joan, a friend of the mother of the groom, wears a bright pink blouse and says she doesn't understand why anyone would want to rebel against their mother, but she'd be willing to learn. She wants to know if I'll be studying lesbian hair. Her daughter is a lesbian, and is often pointing out to her that what we think is feminine and important is generally dictated by the patriarchal portion of our society. Then Joan gets brave, surrounded by all of these laughing rebels, and she asks if I'll be talking to electrologists. She'd had a couple of hairs on her chin—like Leslie's—and she'd gone to the electrologist, who "took care of" them. This woman, an expert, had told her that some women have much more hair on their face. And, also, some women have hair on their nipples. "Think how that must hurt, to have those removed." Joan crosses her arms in front of her pink blouse. She laughs a nervous laugh and her glasses slide up her nose. "I think I'd just have to live with those!"

Gillette Mach 3, $5.99

In Michelle's favorite secret fantasy, she visits all of the friends who know her as Michael, and they welcome her with wry humor and open arms. She imagines going to her usual pub, around the corner from the Chelsea apartment she shares with her wife and two sons, and Henry, the bartender, shaking his head with a smile. "Don't tell me you're gonna have a White Russian," he growls, and that's the end of it. When she's feeling pragmatic, she actually starts to imagine how to accomplish this introduction of herself to the people who have known her the longest. What she wants most is for them to *see* her dressed as Michelle, with her black bobbed wig and black wool dress, rather than for Michael to simply tell them about her. Right now, she's speculating about the possibilities of a mass mailing. "I sent a postcard of my kids last Christmas," she says, only half-joking.

In reality, though, Michelle is only Michael's nighttime persona, a real but sequestered presence who owns a sequined flapper dress and slips into their apartment building when his wife is away with the kids. Her clothes are in garment bags and her corsets and hose are stuffed in the backs of drawers. Although her wife and a couple of close friends know of her existence, dressing and going out are things she does alone or with other transgendered friends. Michelle likes crossing borders and boundaries, pushing the limits and discovering new territory, and, truly, she's not sure how open she wants Michelle's life to be: she freezes when her boys' baby-sitter points out cross-dressers on the Cuban version of *Jenny Jones*, yet shrugs when it is clear the baby-sitter has done the laundry and separated Michelle's underwear from her wife's. "She knows my wife isn't a forty." She imagines telling all of her friends, but then admits she's glad her building doesn't have a doorman. "I'm on the co-op board," she says.

Part of her ambivalence reflects the struggle she's having with her wife, who dealt with her husband's cross-dressing with an out-of-sight, out-of-mind approach until, a year after telling her, Michelle used a whole pack of razors and shaved off most of her body hair, leaving only a small triangle of pubic hair. "It was a flash," Michelle says now, her eyes wide with the memory, "a whole lifetime of sensations that disappeared in adolescence." She recognized that she was taking a drastic step, a step that would effect Michael's existence, too, but it was right before Halloween, and she justified it as a holiday lark. "That's the biggest step you can take," she admits, knowing that body hair is a basic public signal of masculinity. "The minute you shave and you go to your gym, your friend says, 'What the fuck?' " Ironically, when Michelle continued, it won her a measure of respect at her gym, where she works out as Michael, and where a hairless chest signals a serious commitment to developing visibly well-defined muscles. One trainer complimented her for being "cut." But her wife reacted with vehemence and, finally, an ultimatum: no more shaving.

Michelle tried to comply, but felt like she was missing something important when she stopped shaving. She used clippers, easing the setting down shorter and shorter, but in the end, those legalistic distinctions helped neither Michelle nor her wife. "Hair keeps you from feeling," she argues. Her black eyeliner, which rings her eye in an old-fashioned sort of way, helps make her look both serious and seductive, like she knows what she's talking about. She and her wife have reached a stalemate and have returned to a therapist they used to see. For now, they remain locked in limbo, both wanting to please, but not seeing any way to compromise. Her wife is away for a couple of weeks now, and Michelle seems both relieved to postpone decisions and impatient to enjoy her body. She doesn't want to lose her wife, but she doesn't want to be hairy, either.

Compared to this shaving question, Michelle's other forays into public life were simple. After months spent agonizing over catalogue orders, Michelle finally ventured into a Victoria's Secret store. She had planned an excuse, but in the end it seemed lame and unnecessary. "I'm buying this for my sister, she lives in Canada," she says, straightfaced, to an imaginary saleswoman. "They don't have bras over there." Today, she is at once intransigent and sympathetic. She understands at least a little of her wife's dilemma. Shaving brings Michelle's existence home to Michael's bed, making it impossible for her wife to ignore. "Michelle is *out*. My wife's discovered the other woman, and the other woman is me." Michelle laughs silently at the irony of cheating on her wife with herself, but she can't laugh too hard because ultimately, it's true: Michelle is Michael's other love, the woman to whom he is closest.

For a cross-dresser like Michelle, the old distance between appearance and reality has grown thorny and treacherous. First and foremost, drag is a triumph of surface over substance, the suspension of biological belief in favor of a sartorial logic that is skin deep by definition. So surfaces are essential: they are the screens onto which Michelle projects an alternative reality; they are also a dangerously thin veneer, easily punctured by sharp-edged stubble that pushes up from below. Years ago, Michael wore a beard and thought that it was a sign of his leftist politics, a rejection of conservative grooming habits. Looking back, Michelle thinks it was an attempt to hide his transgendered ego behind a mask of masculine hair growth. Smooth skin and a clear window might have been what Michael feared back then, but it is all that Michelle craves now. Since she started shaving again this past spring, her wife has been on a "sex strike," and Michelle's frustration has hardened into longing for "someone who is accepting"—probably, someone who isn't her wife. Shaving, says Michelle, rejecting both compromise and stubble, "is something I have to do."

In the meantime, Michelle has her own theories about slick and smooth, and why it is the rage. She sees the waxed chests of hetero guys at her gym, fortysomething and over, and thinks that *Star Trek* is behind it somehow, the past and the future converging at once. These men are turning their flesh into the spandex of *Deep Space Nine*, smooth and shiny and plasticine. And, at the same time, they are returning to their earliest days, when their bodies were contained by hairless baby skin and their nourishment came from a round smooth breast. Perhaps they use Gillette's latest Mach 3 as Michelle does—in the ads, as sleek and fast as a stealth bomber sliding along a night sky; in fact, a safety razor sold at Rite Aid for $5.99. Michelle is talking about surface, the surface of her body becoming the battlefield for her marriage, and she poses a challenge for herself: "Are you going to burn that bridge or blow it up behind you?" I want to ask if there's anything smoother, slicker, or colder than ice, but I don't.

Disposable Blades, $1.29–$6.99

It took time for what would become the single most important invention for home hair removal to penetrate the American market. King Camp Gillette launched the safety razor with disposable blades in 1895, hoping to capitalize on the increasing popularity of the smooth male chin, but it wasn't until after the century turned that the idea of easy self-grooming began to take hold. In 1903, Gillette sold only fifty-one razors and 168 blades; but in 1904, ninety thousand razors and twelve million blades flew off the shelves. It was a good omen: now, in the late 1990s, the wet-shaver market is worth over one billion dollars, and Gillette manufactures six of the top ten disposable razors. Attracted first to the installation of masculine shaving habits in the privacy of one's home, where an easily purchased safety razor made economic and hygienic sense, feminine fashion has since divided the home shaver market into gendered camps of pink and blue. Daisy double blades might work exactly like Gillette's Goodnews, but color coding is a marketing hint many of us heed: blue razors perch on the sink, pink in the shower stall. Technological advances—the "floating" double blades of the Sensor Excel, for example—are meant for the tough contours of the male chin, whereas design advances—the easy-grip base of the snazzy Sensor—are for the elegant slopes of the female leg.

The most accessible and affordable home depilatory option, razors are a special instrument for teenage girls. They answer a certain necessity born of hormonal maturity (hair) and require a certain operative skill that is easily—but not too easily—grasped and proudly displayed. Like tampons and deodorant, they are the hygienic equipment of adulthood, and are wielded with a public familiarity that betrays itself immediately: cuts and scars are badges of an initiation that few truly want to skip. Many of the girls I spoke to professed ambivalence, even nonchalance, about hair removal and the razors they use, and yet none have eschewed the practice entirely. Like certain other grooming rituals—makeup, for example—that are not connected to the actual health and well-being of body tissue, shaving is a measured choice for most girls, a decision to present their body to the public in a particular way, according to particular standards.

When she was in sixth grade, Josephine Ferorelli, now a Trinity tenth-grader, and her friends were in such a rush toward womanhood, they lied about having their periods and coolly displayed raised white bumps on their legs—battle scars from the hair wars. Josephine's mother warned her it would be a pain to maintain, but Josephine was dying, then, to follow her best friend's lead. She was beginning to feel self-conscious about her legs—suddenly, it seemed, there was hair on them. "Of course then I totally screwed it up," she says. The hair had been soft and light, and then she had shaved and it began to grow stiffer and thicker. At camp, where girls shaved in groups around a communal bucket of water, because privacy was not the point and "there was no bathroom anyway," Josephine used a Gillette Sensor, a typical woman's razor with a wavy blue center, ridged so you won't lose your grip leaning over in the shower. Back then, your choice of razor was as important as your choice of jeans. Josephine remembers the pressure a little shyly, with perhaps less distance than she would like. "You had to be femme—and your razor had to be femme, too."

This "femme" business was, and is, the essence of the problem: Josephine is trying to resist what she calls a "*YM* sense of hygiene"—an approach to women's bodies governed by magazines like *YM* and *Seventeen*, where conquering beauty beasts like fat, acne, and unwanted hair becomes a moral triumph. "I'm still struggling with a warped sense of body image," says Josephine, who hunches a little behind the table but speaks clearly and distinctly, in full adult sentences. "It's so easy to take for granted that you have to fit this generic mold." It's so easy, she means, to believe that it is only thin girls with well-behaved blond hair, perky noses, flashy smiles, and clean-shaven legs that are pretty. Depilation is an essential ingredient, admits Josephine, because "everything else is considered unclean." She knows the drill and can recite the credo, but she's already developed an intellectual's skepticism. "I couldn't tell you why it's important," she says.

And yet, while Josephine works with a schoolgirl's diligence to maintain her intellectual distance from both beauty fads and stereotypes, their logic and sway are hard to resist. In Paris with her mother, brother, and a friend for the summer, Josephine admits she shaved a couple of times, "because it was hot, and I was going to wear shorts, and I like to keep my politics to myself." As far as Josephine's concerned, the aesthetics of body hair removal are in the eye of the beholder, and that's what makes her choices so frustrating. Though she doesn't like participating in a beauty system that she considers sexist, patriarchal, and overly materialistic, she doesn't feel entirely comfortable rejecting it either. She worries that if she has hairy legs, people will assume she "sings folk music." "By not conforming to one stereotype,

I'm conforming to another that others don't like. I wouldn't have such a problem with it if it wasn't such a negative thing in everyone else's eyes." Josephine sighs and utters that timeless schoolgirl's lament: "The guys at my school are just so pathetic."

Slightly older than Josephine, but no less ambivalent, a group of seniors from the Brearley School on Manhattan's Upper East Side remembers their eighth-grade year, when one of the prettiest, most popular girls in their class let her leg hair grow in thick and full. No one in this group was close to this renegade, so they can't report what she was thinking when she made such a controversial decision, but they can describe the scene vividly—a tall blond girl nonchalantly twirling leg hair around her finger in French class. I ask if it was because she was so popular that this girl could get away with something that other girls would not even dare to try. Hooting, shouting, they set me straight. "*No one* got away with it!"

Leg hair, armpit hair, shaving—by now they're used to it, and like jaded veterans, often let it go for months, all winter even, hidden beneath the denim and wool of cool weather fashions. They say it's not important, that it's okay whatever you do, but the truth is they watch it like hawks, carefully recounting their own depilatory evolution, checking the stats to update each other's. Natalie worked this summer at an earthy camp where most of the counselors didn't shave, so she didn't either. Lovingly, playfully, she grew her leg hair, and when she returned to New York, she trumpeted her success to all of her friends, begging them to admire her accomplishment on the first day of preseason practice for field hockey. It is Josie, another member of this group, who laughs as she relays this story, while Natalie sits, a little sheepish, at the opposite end of the couch. None of them, it seems, were as impressed with Natalie's leg hair as Natalie was. They told her, with the bluntness of good friends, to shave it off, it was gross; their hockey coach told her to get rid of it. The final word rested with Natalie's mother, though, who told her that she couldn't go out to dinner with the family unless she shaved.

One thing is immediately and abundantly clear: body hair is not private business. It is, as Josephine says, a matter of projections and impressions. It is the way you choose to face the world, and unfortunately, the world is not made up of understanding girls, who know that not shaving might just be a matter of timing, and not of political preferences. A guy who notices a girl didn't shave for a pool party might think she is, according to this group, "gross" or "gay." Natalie met her summer boyfriend, Eric, who is really cute and not very smart, when she had already decided not to shave; aware of this, she felt obligated to continue through the whole summer. Otherwise, it would have been unfair, like changing the rules midgame.

This group has heard of other depilatory methods, but they are themselves quite dedicated to the ease and convenience of the disposable razor. Other depilatory adventures have proven painful and problematic. Lindsay keeps her curly red hair in a ponytail unless she has blown it straight and is sure she can control it. She advocates shaving as a social nicety, a "courtesy to others." Her experiments with her mother's Epilady were so painful that she steered clear of her mother's bathroom, the scene of the crime, for two full months. Everyone agrees that shaving above the knee is a no-no, though they're not sure why—"it's something social," thinks Josie, linking it somehow to the age-old prohibitions against kissing in bathing suits and sitting on public toilet seats. Natalie reports that she waxes "when it's convenient," and it's really "one of the most painful things." A few minutes later, she blurts that in addition to her legs and bikini area, she's also waxed her mustache, and the raucous conversation sort of tumbles to a stop. No one says, "me too," or "ouch," or anything and Natalie is suddenly shy, keeping quiet until Josie asks why people pay so much money for someone to pour hot wax on their legs. "You could buy CDs with that money," she reasons. "It's good money!" Besides, she wonders, how would she ask her dad to pay for a bikini wax?

A few weeks later, I talk to Suzanne, a junior at a private girls' school in upstate New York, who is tall and tanned and parks her Saab at an angle in her family's driveway. She stopped shaving her leg hair one year, just between soccer season and basketball season, and all she can say is that it was, in the end, "pretty scary." She knows girls who don't shave, and one who doesn't need to, but like Josephine, Josie, Lindsay, Natalie, and their friends, she thinks that it's risky business, letting yourself grow out like that. The reason is short, simple, and clear. She looks away and shrugs, maybe because she thinks it's not what I want to hear. "For girls, body hair isn't good."

A Coda: Revlon Slant-Tipped Tweezers, $3.99

My friend keeps her best tweezers in her pocket, and when her boyfriend stops the car she whips them out and starts plucking in the rearview mirror. It embarrasses him, this compulsion of hers, but she can't help it. It seems terribly important that the stray hairs around her eyebrows be kept in check. She's spoken to her mother, a therapist, about this habit, but it hasn't helped. The prognosis isn't good, she reports. Her mother says it's a disease.

Five

Sheitl Mayses (Wig Stories)

*And the priest shall set the woman before the Lord, and unbind the
hair of the woman's head, and place in her hands the cereal offering
of remembrance, which is the cereal offering of jealousy.*

—Numbers 5:18

For her birthday, Georgie Klein is treating herself to a
haircut by Frederic Fekkai. She has driven to Manhattan
from Brooklyn in her new Jeep—another birthday present to herself—and now she is sitting in Fekkai's busy
new salon above Chanel, sipping espresso and waiting for
this three-hundred-dollar experience to begin. Fekkai
himself comes over, eventually, and begins to arrange her
hair, his eyes on the mirror in front of her. His expression
serious, he fans her hair over her shoulders and watches it
fall; he feels the ends between his fingers. "Just a second,"
she says, holding up her hand to stop him. As if in a
movie—a sci-fi thriller, where nothing is as it first
seems—she reaches up and removes the hair he has been

touching. Fekkai is startled; he hadn't suspected that it was a wig. Georgie smiles a coy, slightly apologetic smile. She loves that her wig is distinctly unwiglike, made of smooth, long, auburn layers that swing across her shoulders—just like her own hair. And she loves that outside the orthodox community of Borough Park, Brooklyn, where she is a well-known *sheitl makher*, or wig dresser, she looks like any other Fekkai customer in a Norma Kamali suit.

Accustomed to eccentricity and well aware that the sensitive core of his business is the customer's ego, Fekkai recovers quickly, though for a moment it looked like he might be annoyed. "Now you're talking," he says, and nods at Georgie in the mirror. For another few seconds he combs her hair with his fingers, nodding slowly to himself in the mirror. Finally, he seems to have decided something, though he's said nothing to Georgie, and he signals to one of the many staff members who hover on the sidelines of the bustling salon floor wearing matching smocks and waiting to escort customers to their shampoo or to summon the makeup artist, who wanders from station to station with a basket of goodies, all for sale.

Returned from her shampoo, performed by yet another salon elf, Georgie is ready for Fekkai, but he is not ready for her. He is at a station diagonally across from Georgie's, and he smiles conspiratorially while he snips away at another woman's hair—hair that is gray and very thin on top and which Georgie can't help mentioning when Fekkai returns. "Why don't you recommend to her a wig?" she asks him, unconsciously marking herself with a Yiddish syntax and a quiet Hungarian inflection. She's eager for him to see her as a colleague, and for his approval of her wig, but Fekkai just shrugs and lets his smile settle on her in the mirror. Part Vietnamese, part Egyptian, and part French, he is extremely handsome, with dark almond eyes, healthy olive skin, and a flash of black hair that waves low across his forehead; his attention is enough for now.

When her cell phone rings he grabs it from the counter, opens it, and hands it to her without missing a beat; nothing is a distraction here. He snips away quickly and confidently while she converses quietly for only a moment. Elie Wiesel has canceled his date to speak at a benefit she is organizing for Israeli orphans. Her eyes flicker over Fekkai for a moment then settle on me. "Do you know anyone famous?" she asks.

Finally, he is finished. "Are you going to put that back on?" Fekkai asks, pointing to Georgie's wig, which is lying on the counter between a jar of combs and Georgie's tiny phone. He is reluctant to style her hair—or, rather, to have one of his staff style it—if she is going to crush it under the wig. But Georgie herself is reluctant to give up even an ounce of this experience.

"Just do what you're going to do," she tells him, urging him to style it as he would any other customer's hair. When he hesitates, she turns to me, wondering how we can convince him to style her hair without promising that she'll leave off her wig. Like her customers, Georgie has worn a wig for all of her married life, so that her hair is shielded from the gaze of men who are not her husband, and her business depends on her reputation as a *frum*, or pious, woman. Even a short adventure in naked hair would be taking a big risk—it's probably risky just being here, allowing Fekkai and anyone else here to see her without her wig. Georgie returns his gaze in the mirror, challenging him, and finally, Fekkai loses his nerve. He starts to style her hair.

For Jewish men, covering the head is a matter of pious custom, a way of showing that you are humble, beneath the gaze of the One above. For Jewish women, it is a different matter, bound up in the knotty ties among sexuality, transgression, and subjection. In the hazing ritual prescribed for adulterous wives in Numbers, the suspected *sotah* (errant wife) is first plied with written accusations of her affair, then brought before the presence of the Lord, and the presiding priest is authorized to *porah et rosh ha'ishah*, or expose her hair. After ingesting the "bitter water" used to wash the print from her husband's accusation, a mysterious alchemical reaction will prove her guilt, swelling her body, causing her great pain, and rendering her an "execration among her people." This elaborate test and the vagueness of her punishment are necessitated by the absence of witnesses to her crime; an adulterous wife who was seen committing her crime was stoned to death, unless she was the wife of a priest—then she was burned.

The exact meaning of *porah* remains unclear. Some claim it means to expose the hair, others that it is more precise, meaning to dishevel, or unbraid the hair. Nor is the role of this step in the investigation of the sotah entirely obvious either. Certainly, it dramatized her subjection to the priest and her husband's suspicions. It also seems to have been a moment of humiliation for her, perhaps even a violation. But did it also brand her with the mark of her alleged indiscretion, imprinting an indelible image of sexual voraciousness on the minds of her accusers? As with many Biblical punishments, the hair ritual of the sotah investigation now seems to make perfect retaliatory sense. When the French courts did not work fast or effectively enough at the end of World War II, angry citizens knew exactly what to do with suspected female collaborators; they shaved their heads and walked them through the streets.

Puzzling though it was, the process of discovering the guilt of suspected sotah made sense to the Talmudic rabbis, too. In their explicatory endeavors, they were able to read between the lines of the Numbers passage to find the Biblical root, and thus the religious rationale, for what became the Talmudic consensus on *pe'ah nakhrit*, or women's hair covering. Since an adulterous, immodest women is punished by having her hair exposed, the rabbis reasoned that a modest virtuous woman must be required by God to do the opposite, to keep her hair hidden. By the early years of the Christian period, rabbinic authority had agreed that married women were to keep their hair completely covered in public, and that it was forbidden for men to pray in the exposed presence of hair that was usually covered. "The sight of a woman's hair constitutes an erotic stimulus," the Talmud states flatly. Her duty to keep it hidden protected the essential fabric of Jewish society: the woman's virtue, the husband's prerogative, the exclusivity of the family unit, and the sanctity of prayer. Tertullian, Roman emperor at the turn of the second century C.E., recorded the success of the rabbinical teachings, noting that "among the Jews, it is so usual for their women to have their head veiled that this is the means by which they may be recognized."

Far from being frustrated by the enigmatic omissions of the sotah passage, the Talmudic rabbis and their successors seem to have turned vagueness to advantage. Although the prohibition on exposing one's hair to public view had its origins in the Bible, in practice its force comes less from *dat moshe*, the laws of Moses, and more from what has come to be called *dat yehudit*, the customs of the Jews. Having been explicated by the rabbis and reinforced by centuries of practical adherence, pe'ah nakhrit carries the weight of God through the blood and voice of the ancestors. It is repeated, almost without variance, in code after code of Jewish law. A sixth-century commentary on Genesis urges *all* women to cover their heads, "like one who commits a crime and is abashed by it in the presence of people." And the *Shulkhan Arukh*, a sixteenth-century text that has become a standard for post-Talmudic religious observance, echoes the rabbis without question. "It is forbidden to gaze upon a woman's beauty," it states, "or to stare at women washing clothes. . . . One may not hear them sing or see their hair."

Using anecdote to tender the fruits of restraint and humility, the Talmud relates several tales that join feminine virtue to hair modesty. For instance: Rachel, the wife of Rabbi Akiba, martyred muse of the Talmudic rabbis, was disowned by her family when she married

Akiba, then a lowly shepherd employed by her wealthy father. Her only condition to the marriage was that Akiba devote his life to Torah study. This he did, forcing her to support them with any means she could muster. The resourceful Rachel sold her hair, proclaiming to all the world that Torah and husband come before vanity, pride, and the private significance of a married woman's hair. Husbands who don't mind their wives going about with uncovered hair, claims the Talmud, are likely not to mind other violations of proper decorum as well, such as bare arms and bathing and "acting frivolously with other men." Such lax and apathetic husbands are to be condemned along with their wives, since they are like men who find a fly in their bowl and, after removing it, eat the soup anyway.

And yet, despite the confident interpretations of the Talmudic rabbis and the constant reinforcement of their successors, the murkiness of the biblical passage has not been completely dispelled. Various sages have wondered, for instance, if unmarried women are included in the prohibition; and though most agree that they are not, doubts persist—might they be? The exact boundaries of public space have caused difficulty, too: is the courtyard of a woman's own home "public," and in what category are her husband's eyes—are they public? Rabbi Judah, student of Rabbi Akiba, worries aloud in the Talmud that pe'ah nakhrit might not go far enough to dissolve the corruptive power of exposed female locks, since the ritual exposure of the sotah's hair could arouse and corrupt the impressionable young priests assigned to unbind it.

When the sages asked Kimhit, mother of seven sons, all of whom became high priests, how she had merited such a blessing, she attributes her good fortunes to the virtue of her hidden hair. "The walls of my house have never seen the hairs of my head," she tells the rabbis. But the rabbis are not so easily convinced. Many women, they tell her, can say this about themselves. They wondered: what else makes you special?

An Ashkenazi Jew born just after World War II in Budapest, Hungary, Georgie arrived in the United States in 1963, just two days before John F. Kennedy was shot and killed in Dallas. Her father, a former factory worker, had had a stroke before the family left Hungary; by the time they settled in the Williamsburg section of Brooklyn and Georgie's mother found work in the box factory that still employs her, he needed constant care at home. "My sister was brilliant," says Georgie, "so I stayed." While caring for her father, Georgie drew and practiced the latest hairstyles on her neighbors. At fifteen, she went to Robert Fiance Beauty School in Manhattan, and at sixteen, she opened her own shop. She became a sheitl makher only gradually, as her young customers began to get married and wear wigs.

Even now, when Georgie wigs are worn all over the world and people travel from as far away as Australia and Switzerland to have Georgie style their wigs—even now, Georgie wants it made clear that she was a hairdresser before she was a wig dresser. Though she is fully ensconced in this religious world—she is herself a religious person—it cannot completely contain her. In a neighborhood where many women never learn to drive, Georgie roars down the streets in her white Jeep, her cell phone pinned between her shoulder and her ear. And in a world where it is considered a great privilege for a woman to be able to stay at home with her children, Georgie is the highly visible helm of a hugely successful business. Her three-story building on Sixteenth Avenue in Borough Park contains shops, a café, and a banquet hall. The wig salon and its winter garden take up the third floor, and city councilman Noach Dear, Borough Park's answer to the Reverend Al Sharpton, rents space on the second.

Visibility and power—two things that an orthodox woman, especially in a traditional community like Borough Park, are not supposed to have. But Georgie seems unafraid of the midtown crowds as she walks out onto Fifty-seventh Street, her wig curling on her shoulders, just like her hair did a few minutes ago when Fekkai finished drying and arranging it so that it looked, to me, much the same as it did before he began. Far from being disappointed, Georgie received Fekkai's syles as if it were a tribute; obviously, the famous man thought she was doing the right thing. Unlike many of her clients, whose hair is also covered all the time, protected from the sun but also pinned next to the head, Georgie keeps her hair thick and shiny. She wears it proudly, if only in private, coloring it to create the highlights the sun can't, and conditioning it with seaweed so that it isn't damaged from the friction of her wig. It is an emblem of her skill, a hidden badge of distinction that earns her envious glances whenever, in the feminine security of her shop, she removes the covering that mimics it so perfectly.

We walk over to Henri Bendel, where Georgie buys a black jersey top for $295 without trying it on. In the upstairs café we order coffee, and wait for the saleswoman to bring Georgie's top and her charge card over. When I ask Georgie what would have happened if she'd given in to Fekkai and gone without her wig, she shrugs and sighs. "Someone is always criticizing me for something," she says.

In the Long Island town of Lawrence where Debbie lives, only a handful of the married orthodox women wear wigs. Most don't cover their hair, but for those who do, hats are their covering of choice. "Berets," says one woman, who wears her two wigs only on special occasions. "That's the secret. You don't look too conspicuous."

Conspicuous is exactly what religious Jewish women do not want to be. But "blending in" is not always easy, especially since their community is only a small enclave in a larger, more dynamic, multicultural setting. Religious women take special care not to distance themselves from their peers. On the streets of Borough Park, the possibilities of fashion have been converted to a sense of uniformity, where rules of modesty and very real physical and cultural isolation have combined to limit the styles that women will wear: navy blue and hunter green are the colors the season I visit, and skirt lengths are on the short side, falling midcalf over seamed stockings that everybody wears because that's what their mothers and grandmothers wore in Europe. They are honestly surprised, perhaps even secretly pleased, to hear that a black seam running up the back of a woman's calf is a staple image of magazine erotica. "*Hot?*" They repeat skeptically, "These are *hot?*"

But in places like Lawrence, where the orthodox community prides itself on its modernity, and where Jewish isolation is neither possible nor desirable, anxiety turns more toward the world at large. Modern orthodox women have access to television, magazines, stores—all of the major repositories of American beauty norms. But they also have certain religious pressures to contend with, a knowledge of custom and codes that, no matter what they decide, makes innocence impossible.

Debbie has come to Georgie's with her fiancé's sister, her future sister-in-law, Batya. Heavy, big-busted, with a wide face and a custom sheitl made of European hair and cut in a long, layered style almost exactly like Georgie's own, Batya is emphatic about everything. "I *love* this sheitl," she says, brushing her wig in front of the mirror at Georgie's work station. "It's the best investment I *ever* made."

Debbie is tall, blond, and quiet. While Batya talks, Debbie's mouth purses around her teeth, as if she wants to say something, but can't quite find the courage. It's clear that Batya is running the show. While Georgie works on someone else, Batya sits Debbie down at a nearby station. First, though the color is all wrong, Batya wants Debbie to try on her wig. Unlike cheaper wigs, it is made from European hair—as opposed to synthetic or Asian hair that has been chemically lightened and curled. And it is also custom-made, designed by Georgie and hand-sewn by a Hungarian wig maker in Brooklyn whose identity is guarded as a potentially lethal trade secret.

With Batya's full wig over her thick hair, Debbie looks like a child playing dress-up. The wig is too dark, too thick, and too big for Debbie's head. She looks at herself skeptically in the mirror, and her chin wrinkles; she's trying her best not to cry. Batya, convinced that all Debbie needs is for the wig to match her color, is combing Debbie's hand through the back of the wig. "Did you ever see such beautiful hair in your life?" she asks Debbie. Debbie answers, softly, with a question. "Can I try a fall?" She wants to try to wear a hairpiece, instead of a full wig. Certain American rabbis have said that it is okay for a woman to show a narrow band of hair at the forehead, and Debbie is imagining that with her own hair showing in front, she will look almost exactly as she does without the wig.

While Yolanda, Georgie's assistant, goes in search of a blond fall, Georgie tries to convince Debbie that she is better off wearing a wig. Falls sit too far back on the head, Georgie tells her, and are uncomfortable and inconvenient. "It's too hard to wear," Georgie tells her, balancing Batya's outsized voice with her own quiet, inflected English. "You'll hate me in two weeks if you get the fall."

Finally, Debbie is convinced. The fall is heavy and doesn't blend well with her hair: Debbie's hair has an ashy cast to it, while the blonde of the fall is gold in tone; her hair hangs very straight, and the bouncy bulk of the fall keeps it from actually blending with her own hair. Reluctantly, she hands the fall back to Yolanda and allows Batya to sit her in

Georgie's chair to be fitted for the cap, or foundation, of her custom wig.

"I'm not sure I'm going to cover," Debbie whispers beneath the clatter of Batya's and Georgie's voices. She won't say anything more about it, and sits in silence as Georgie wraps her head tightly in plastic wrap and then criss-crosses it with Scotch tape—this will be the "mold" for her foundation. Georgie understands Debbie's anxieties and leaves room at the front of the cap so that Debbie's own hair can be combed back and over the front of the wig. She'll be able to keep her natural hairline after all.

"I'm counting my blessings," Georgie says, as she carefully draws an inch or so of Debbie's hair from under the front of the Saran Wrap cap. "If you would be Hasidic, we'd have a problem." Batya, not sure that Debbie understands, translates for her. "If you would be *Hasidische*," she says, using the Yiddish adjective instead of the English, "you'd have to have *every strand* covered. Your wig would be down here." Debbie's hairline is relatively close to her brows, and both Georgie and Batya know that it's very uncomfortable to have a wig sitting so low. "In the summer, you would *die*."

After she is fitted for her cap, Debbie sits on a stone bench in the solarium and stares at the Greek columns, properly decrepit, that are painted on the rag-rolled walls, while Georgie and Batya use the natural light to match her hair to hair that will be used for the wig. From a box full of blond ponytails, most of which came from Italy and Belgium, Georgie finds hair that matches Debbie's lightest highlights, but she doesn't have any to match the ashy undertones. Debbie winces when Georgie bends her head forward and snips off a little chunk of her hair so that Sara, Georgie's hair buyer, can take it with her later in the week when she goes to see Miriam, a hair importer in Borough Park. "Don't worry," Georgie says briskly. "No one will notice. You can't see a thing."

Later, Batya tells me that her brother, Debbie's fiancé, is encouraging her not to cover her hair. "He's just trying to bug our mother," Batya says, looking annoyed. "He's never had to work a day in his life. He's very spoiled." She starts to grin. "But he is a *knock-out.*" Debbie's own mother, whom Batya dismisses as a "Mercedes-driving, smoking, thin-as-a-rail blond," doesn't cover her hair either, though, and Batya's mother is a little worried that Debbie will not follow through. "My mother is *plotzing*," says Batya. "I tell her not to worry—Debbie will wear the wig. She's a good girl."

But the next day, just before the plastic bag containing the mold for Debbie's cap goes to the custom cap maker in Borough Park, Debbie calls and tells Georgie not to send it. She's not ready to commit to the wig.

Borough Park is a neighborhood of dense contradiction. Despite the promise of its name, it boasts only a couple of concrete playgrounds and a random lawn or two; there are no parks to speak of in Borough Park. It is the home of more than a hundred thousand individuals housed in two-hundred square blocks, but only two visible sets of women: those who cover their hair and those who do not. Those who do, of course, are Jewish, members of one of the

Hasidic sects based in the area—Bobov, Gribov, Ger, Spinka, or Belz, who moved into the neighborhood in the 1950s and sixties as the Irish moved out—or of another orthodox group, most of whom are traditional, not modern. The women who do not cover their hair are black, Polish, or part of a growing Hispanic minority; their presence is marked not only by their hair, but by their flesh. Even in summer, the Jewish women wear long sleeves, stockings, hats. In contrast, the non-Jews look naked. The boundaries that separate the different groups—all of whom live and work in close proximity, and yet never seem to meet on the street—are made of muscle, bone, tendon, and tissue. The exposed hair, arms, and bellies of the non-Jews speak not just of differences in fashion and preference, or even in religion and practice. It seems, to an outsider, that it is the boldness in the step of the Polish girls' naked legs that the Jewish women lack.

It is because of the uniformity of the Jewish women's couture—their long, pleated skirts, their wigs and colored straw hats—that Tillie and Malka stand out in the kosher pizza place on Sixteenth Avenue. They are seated at a table in the front, speaking in Yiddish about vacations in their youth. But unlike anyone else around them who might conduct a conversation in Yiddish, they are dressed in stretch pants and T-shirts, and their thin hair is completely uncovered. It sparkles under the fluorescent lights. Both of them came from Poland after the war, and on their arms I can see the searing blue ink of concentration camp numbers. They have taken the subway from the Lower East Side of Manhattan to Borough Park to see a travel agent; this summer, they are going back to Poland for the first time.

In the old country, Tillie's grandmother was a renowned sheitl makher, and she tells without irony the apocryphal legend of her success. When her daughter married, she made her a wig so beautiful, so refined, that her friends were scandalized the day after the girl's wedding. "Isn't your daughter going to wear a wig?" they asked Tillie's grandmother. Even her closest friends had been fooled by so fabulous a wig.

Tillie herself owns two wigs, both of which she only wears for weddings, funerals, and her occasional trips to the synagogue. When she first arrived here, she notes, American Jews didn't wear wigs at all. She attributes the sheitl revival of the late-1950s and 1960s to the postwar influx of Hungarian Jews. "They were very religious," she says knowingly. And then, as if she's just begun to make the connection: "You know, the Hungarians were only one year in the concentration camps. Only one year. We went in 1941; they went in 1944." Perhaps, she is implying, in that one year the Hungarians did not experience enough terror to lose their faith in God—or in the protective covering of the sheitl.

When Malka goes to synagogue—which is infrequently—she wears a hat. She's never owned a wig, and neither did her mother. In fact, the whole concept makes her impatient. "I was liberated *before* the war," she says, gripping my arm with her nails to make sure I understand.

Tillie is unperturbed by her friend's implied criticism. She clutches her purse and Malka's arm as they step out onto the busy sidewalk. "If my parents would live," she says with a shrug, "I would wear a wig. But Hitler killed them, so what good is it?"

∞

Among Holocaust survivors in New York, the war has its own cosmic geography. First is *before the war*: no matter if life was tough and dirty, stunted by anti-Semitism and poverty, *before the war* was a good time, the normal time against which all other times must be judged. Then, *the camps*: Hell. The fire through which survivors walked, stumbling and lost, until they somehow, miraculously, ended up on the other side. Next, *the DP camps*: a misplaced limbo, a purgatory after the fact. It is here, in the Displaced Persons camps, that the postwar lives of many New York survivors began to take shape. They talk about the DP camps like Baby Boomers talk about college and California: this is where my journey of self-discovery began to bear fruit; this is where I found my husband, my wife, my career.

For Claire Grunwald, it was where she learned to make wigs. "We were living pretty comfortably, considering," she says of her family's four years in a DP camp outside of Nuremberg, Germany. "They gave us an apartment to ourselves, since we had so many—my mother, myself, and my four sisters. But that's not a life. It's limbo. My mother knew we had to do something." With a mixture of panic, surprise, and entrepreneurial prescience, Claire's aunt had written to her sister in 1938: "There are no sheitl makhers in America." Remembering this seven years later, Claire's mother apprenticed her daughter to a wig maker. For four years, from 1945–49, Claire commuted every day from the DP camp in Furhte to a beauty salon in Nuremberg. While her family waited for the visas that would bring them to America, Claire learned the intricacies of wig making—how to turn, weft, and blend, how to ventilate and sew.

To her infinite pride, she also learned about hair in Nuremberg. For months, her only job was to make sure that all of the hairs in a single batch—each individual hair—were tied at the root and not at the end. Now, with an elfin smile and a finger in the air, she will tell you that this is the secret to her current success; those months she spent sorting (the proper term is "turning") hair in Germany are one of the main reasons the wigs made under her supervision, for her own Claire's Accuhair of Flatbush, are considered by some to be the best in the world. Patiently, in a high, accented voice, Claire will explain that hair must—absolutely must—be tied into the wig the same way it grows on the head. In other words, each individual hair must be connected to the cap at its root, never by the end. If even one hair is wrong, the cuticles that line each hair in the same direction will bristle against each other and cause the hair to knot; the wig will mat and be worthless.

Now that Claire, at sixty-five, owns one of the biggest custom wig businesses in the world, she has her own employees whose only job is to "turn." As she did years ago, they use a wooden stick to agitate batches of hair until any wayward ones—those whose ends lie next to the roots of others—separate themselves from the others and are pulled from the tray.

Claire's aunt's advice proved not only sound, but prophetic. Within a week of her family's arrival in Manhattan's Lower East Side, Claire found employment as a wig maker at a midtown firm called Madame Marie. She made thirty dollars a week. Eventually, she moved to Schwerner and Oppenheim, which occupied the entire floor of a factory building on Twenty-second Street. Young, and skilled in both foundation work and wefting, Claire caused some tension when she began to move up the ladder at Schwerner and Oppenheim. Another Hungarian Jewish woman, thinking she'd been passed over, threatened to quit when Claire began to train as a stylist. And when Claire later returned to the ventilating line for a time, her peers thought her stuck-up.

"Whenever they saw the boss coming, they'd say, 'Clara, don't you have to go to the toilet? Maybe you need a rest.' I thought they were so nice, these girls. But then the boss, he sees I'm not working. So I was laid off," Claire says. And then, leaning in: "Well, I was fired, really."

After that, she made sixty dollars a week slip-stitching silk ties in the garment district. She didn't return to the wig business again until after the birth of her second child, when a series of miscarriages made her look for something to do at home. Now she owns a three-story building on Avenue M in Flatbush, where all phases of the wig business are conducted, from hair sorting to wig styling. Her three daughters, Chaya, Chani, and Silky, as well as her husband, Moishe, work with her, managing this *oytzer*—gold mine— that she has created. Everywhere Claire goes, people recognize her and say hello. Hers is the only wig business in Brooklyn that sells exclusively European hair wigs, most of which are custom-made. She plays Bergdorf's to Georgie's Macy's. When I ask about her competition, Claire just shakes her head and smiles indulgently. "It costs twenty-five to one hundred dollars to manufacture a wig in Korea. They sell it here for two hundred fifty to three thousand dollars. They're making money—why should they bother [to make high-quality custom wigs]? I have no competition, really."

One can usually discern that a woman is wearing a wig, and even if a man cannot tell, in the vast majority of cases, a woman can.

—Rabbi Moshe Feinstein, *Responsa Iggerot Moshe*

Though Jewish women wore wigs and falls in the Talmudic era, they were not used to satisfy the requirement of hiding the hair. The Jewish use of a wig for pe'ah nakhrit is a modern innovation for an ancient custom, and since its inception has been plagued with anxiety. Medieval Jews were distanced from their gentile peers by a series of sartorial distinctions, sometimes voluntary, sometimes imposed, almost continuously observed after the beginning of the twelfth century. When the conical, highly visible *Judenhut*, or Jewish hat, fell into disuse, Christian governments, aided by Papal councils, devised other means for distinguishing Jewish subjects. Beginning in the thirteenth century, a number of European territories required Jewish women to wear a white veil with two blue stripes; in others, a yellow or red badge, round like a donut or star-shaped, was required to be pinned to the breast of Jewish men and women alike. In Marseilles, all Jews over seven years of age were allowed to choose between wearing a yellow badge or a yellow hat. In Italy, the Holy Roman Emperor Frederick II decreed in 1222 that his Jewish subjects should wear the Greek letter *Tau* cut from blue cloth, reminding them of their social status—*last* in the Hebrew alphabet, and in the original Greek alphabet—with a cross.

Medieval dress requirements served the purpose of Jew and gentile alike, despite their often heinous motivation. Christian governments and their citizens felt it necessary to be aware of the Jew, on the street and in business, in order to be prepared for the treachery of which the Jew was always capable. Jews, wary of the motives of their Christian counterparts and committed to the purity of their rituals and their birth, valued their separateness as well as their community's cohesion. Whenever assimilation seemed imminent, Jewish leaders protested the probable decline in traditional observations vociferously, reminding their congregants of the Bible's premonitory admonition to forego *hukkot ha goyem*, the ways of the gentiles. In his *Mishnah Torah*, the Spanish scholar Maimonides cited the Talmud, explicitly recalling that the prohibition included gentile hairstyles.

By the time Moses Mendelssohn uttered his famous dictum of assimilatory compromise, the wig crisis was almost over. "Be a man on the street and a Jew in your tent," he advised his followers in the German Jewish Enlightenment movement of the eighteenth century, articulating a new expanse of fashion possibilities. If allowed by Christian governments, the Jew might decide to dress like any other person; he or she might walk the streets without distinction, and perhaps, without molestation. Taking advantage of the demise of state laws dictating special dress requirements for Jews, many nineteenth-century German Jews followed Mendelssohn's advice and adopted the dress and guise of their gentile peers. But they were not necessarily the pioneers they imagined themselves to be. Along with the implications of Mendelssohn's statement, wigs (sheitls) had already been accepted by the rabbis of Italy, who had come to support the Italian Jewish women's desire to follow the gentile lead and take off the stifling headdresses of medieval modesty. When Rabbi Leon of Modena wrote his *Historia dei Riti Ebraici* in the early seventeenth century, he assured his gentile readers that Jews could indeed adapt to sartorial freedom. "The women also apparel themselves in the habit of the countries where they inhabit," he wrote. "But when they are married, upon their wedding day they cover their own hair, wearing either a perruke or dressing, or some other hair or something else that may counterfeit natural hair . . ."

What Rabbi Leon takes to be a virtue, however, others saw as a dangerous precedent. The wig's ability to "counterfeit natural hair" was precisely what made it objectionable, since the principle of *ma'arit ha-ayin* prohibits Jews from even *seeming* to flout Jewish law. A sixteenth-century rabbinic text addresses the issue, claiming that it makes no difference if the wig is made of hair from another woman, "as long as it is made as a hair covering and is unconnected to her scalp." For most Ashkenazic (German-descended) Jews the question was resolved by the end of the eighteenth century, but the Sephardic (Spanish-descended) rabbinate has never approved of wigs as a suitable head covering. *S'dei Hemed*, a nineteenth-century Sephardic encyclopedia of Jewish law, is blunt in its rejection. "Even if there is no outright prohibition," it states, "it is still improper for married Jewish women to wear wigs in our region. It is immodest, and not for the sake of such women were we redeemed from Egypt."

Ironically, in early twentieth-century America, ma'arit ha-ayin became a moot issue in the sheitl market, where it was a distinct *lack* of verisimilitude that led women to abandon their wigs once they reached the promised land. Even in orthodox circles, wigs fell into disfavor very quickly on this side of the Atlantic. In Hartford, Connecticut, fashion-minded orthodox women found a rabbinic spokesperson in Rabbi Isaac Hurewitz, who provided a Halakhic rationale for their abandonment of the sheitl. Rabbi Hurewitz's reasoning focused on the *Shulkhan Arukh*'s prohibition of men's praying in the presence of "hair that is accustomed to being covered." Both tenacious and reasonable, Rabbi Hurewitz zeroed in on the loophole: is it forbidden to pray in the presence of hair that is *not* customarily covered—like that of twentieth-century American Jewish women? And if it is not forbidden to pray, certainly it cannot be forbidden to conduct lesser business, like walking, eating, or reading.

The chief rabbi of Hartford from 1895 until his death in 1935, Rabbi Hurewitz was a respected Talmudic scholar and authority. Trained in the great European yeshivas and ordained by one of the leading rabbis of the period, Isaac Elchanan Spector, Hurewitz was nonetheless bound to dwell on Earth, in America, at a time when the possibilities of assimilation—at least of *fitting in*—were especially compelling. While not without its anti-Semitic moments, America truly did seem like the land of opportunity, even for those whose orthodoxy distanced them from many of the pleasures of American abundance.

Indeed, Hurewitz's *Yad Halevi* is more striking for its secular anxieties than for its theological reasoning. "If all Jewish women, young and old, are forced to cover their heads with a wig," threatened Rabbi Hurewitz, "it will be a blemish and a mark of scorn in their [the gentile's] eyes, and the [Jewish women] will appear as uncivilized savages who aren't fit to enter the land: similar to the Chinese, who go about with braided hair." As Congress debated immigration quotas—the first sweeping immigration restrictions were passed in the midst of Rabbi Hurewitz's Hartford tenure, in 1921 and 1924—Rabbi Hurewitz worried about the sheitls of those who might want to come to America. If they arrived in wigs, would they be turned back at the gates, like those with glaucoma and consumption?

Of course they weren't, but Rabbi Hurewitz was not alone in his anxiety. Nor was he alone in his dislike of the sheitl aesthetic. In Abraham Cahan's famous story, *Yekl* (the novel that became the movie *Hester Street*), the estrangement of an Americanized husband, Jake, from his fresh-off-the-boat wife, Gitl, is illustrated first by his discomfort with her sheitl. When he pushes her to remove it and she insists on putting on her "Saturday kerchief" in its place, Jake reluctantly shields her from sight in the busy train station with his back, "gnashing his teeth with disgust and shame." Eventually, Gitl sees the error of her ways, trading her sheitl for a smart, *Americanische* hat, and Jake for a nicer guy.

In America, before the war, it was *shver tsu zein a yid*—"hard to be a Jew," and by extension, hard to look like one, so much of Madame Marie's and Schwerner and Oppenheim's clientele came from the theater and the black community, not from among Jews. For those who did wear wigs, it was important then, as it is now, that they look as much like real hair as possible. Before her wedding, in 1952, Claire returned to Schwerner and Oppenheim to purchase two wigs. She paid one hundred and fifty dollars for each of them—"a fortune!"—but they were good quality, and she really didn't have a choice; she didn't even consider not covering her hair. "There was no garbage around then," she says, referring obliquely to the synthetic and Asian hair wigs that are machine wefted in Korea and sold by vendors like Georgie for $150–$400. But still, the thought of wearing a wig outside her orthodox neighborhood in the Bed-Stuy section of Brooklyn was a bit daunting. "Outside, you didn't want anyone to know. I was so careful that no one should see I was wearing a wig."

Though the New York orthodox community itself has changed, becoming more religious, more invested in rules like those regarding hair covering for women, the ambivalence surrounding wigs has not. Statistics say that only thirty-four percent of modern orthodox women cover their hair, but even in communities like Borough Park, where most, if not all, of the women cover their hair, becoming accustomed to wearing a wig is not so easy. On the eve of her wedding, the sister of one young woman I met wrote a letter to her hair, explaining why it could no longer be a part of her public life, apologizing and bidding it farewell.

First-time brides like Debbie are especially nervous, and go to great lengths to find a wig that will approximate, as closely as possible, their own hair's color, texture, and style. It is only later that the women learn to be fond of their wigs, to revel in the freedoms they afford them—the freedom to put on their hair and walk out the door in a matter of minutes, every morning; the freedom to change their hairstyle, or color, or length, with a gesture as simple as changing a shirt. In essence, it is the freedom to buy for yourself what every woman wants: perfect hair.

Thus, the wig culture of orthodox Jews exists at a strange juncture: between the real and the simulated, between tradition and fashion, between ambivalence and aspiration. At a *sheitl yirid* (sale) held on a Sunday morning at the Gribover *Simcha* (party) Hall in Borough Park, the names of styles are scrawled in black marker on the flaps of the cardboard boxes that hold the wigs. Individually, these names are awkward, clumsily translated from Yiddish; they are not alluring or catchy in the way that trademark appellations for mainstream consumer objects are wont to be. But collectively, they are something else, a testimony, perhaps, to ambitions wrought in odd but hauntingly accurate English.

Amid the wigs that lay claim to modernity with names like "E-mail," and "World Wide Web," and those that stake out a classical territory—"Matisse" and "Contessa"—are others that speak to vaguer, hungrier impulses. A group of young women with babies propped on their hips are crowded around a box marked "Sophia the Poet," and a woman and her teenage daughter are going through another containing a number of dark brown wigs called "Like a Taxi II." The mother tells me that they are looking for a wig with lighter highlights than the one she has, for the summer. But it seems that they might just as easily be looking for what the name implies—speed, cunning, mobility, a bright yellow flash with a light on top. A box marked "Greys" stands full and untouched in the center of the room. Unless you had to, would you buy age?

As she must be, Claire is a firm believer in the alternative reality represented by her wigs. When she is stuck, in conversation, she runs her fingers through her hair, scratching them lightly against what would be, if she were not wearing a wig, her scalp. It is a gesture that is second nature to teenage girls, who rely on their hair to say things that they are not able to about themselves. Though modest in her way, Claire has none of the shyness of an adolescent girl. Her gesture is one of faith, a confident demonstration. Look, she is saying, I have great hair. Blond and smooth, styled in a wavy, layered cut that falls softly around her face, her hair is utterly unlike the hair of my other sixty-five-year-old acquaintances. On the surface, at least, it's true: she does have great hair.

Her easy faith in the simulated reality of her wigs, she would have you believe, is evidence of the depth of her religious faith. God created men and women the way they are, all fiery attraction and weak imperfection, and thus necessitated pe'ah nekhrit, the covering of women's hair. And it is God that has made her business successful. "In my wildest dreams, I'm never thinking that I'm going to have a building like I'm having now," she says, taking off her rhinestone glasses so that I can see, in her eyes, how serious she is. "It's all in God's hands."

But to the untrained, or unreligious, eye, it seems a lot is in Claire's hands. Once in a while, when she begins to think about how hard it was for a woman to be taken seriously as a business person, she'll let on that with or without God's help, she has built an extremely successful business out of nothing. Before Chaya became her full-time manager a year or so ago, Claire had been trying to hire a young man to take care of the business end of things. "They didn't understand anything!" she says of the men she hired. "I knew it all. I saw it all. But every time I hired someone, they thought I was stupid like their mothers."

Chaya, however, knows perfectly well that Claire is much smarter than the dull mothers of cocky young men, and the men themselves. In her red suit, white pumps, and layered wig, she has the wiry look of the eighties business woman—efficient, driven, tough. She has three teenaged children of her own, is on her second marriage, and once owned her own Kosher vegetarian catering business, which she ran out of the basement of Claire's house in Flatbush. In charge of overseeing the entirety of her mother's business—except for the accounting, which her father handles—Chaya carries a great deal of responsibility on her thin shoulders. And yet, despite the serious, public nature of her work, when Chaya is with Claire she is very much a daughter.

They wait together, in Claire's office, for Claire's one o'clock appointment. A woman named Esther is coming to pick out the hair for a new, formal wig. At five of one, Chaya calls down to the desk, wondering if Esther has arrived. Not yet, the receptionist tells her, but she has called every day this week to confirm; she is sure she'll come. "We love this woman to death," Chaya says to me. "But she's—"

"Ah, ah!" Claire swivels her chair around and shakes her finger at Chaya.

"I know, I know," Chaya says, acknowledging that she shouldn't be telling a strange writer bad things about a good customer. "But it's just that Esther—"

"Chaya!" Claire warns.

"I was only going to tell her that Esther is wonderful, but—"

"Chaya! You have spoken *loshn hora*!" Claire admonishes, using the Hebrew expression for nasty gossip. Chaya turns bright red. She is suddenly a ten-year-old girl who has been chastised by her mother in front of a stranger. "And I have embarrassed you." Claire turns apologetically and touches Chaya's hand. She concedes, "Esther is a little unreliable." She and Chaya giggle; Claire's lapse into loshn hora suits them both. "I shouldn't have said that, but . . ." Claire is trying to explain why she can do with impunity what her daughter could not. Finally, she's got it. "There's a saying: *Yedem toyer hot a tyrele* . . ."

Chaya translates for me. "Next to every big gate, there is a little door . . ."

Six

So Long as Their Hair Was On

The weak-haired child will remain all its life weak in ambition.
—Charles Nessler, *The Story of Hair*

The western half of Twenty-third Street in Manhattan has a big-avenue feel to it; it is wide and lined with big buildings and is not at all quaint and historic like the other Chelsea streets that run parallel. There are stores, restaurants, apartment buildings terraced with scaffolding, one broad-fronted synagogue—this could be any big city with millions to house, feed, and amuse. This must be why La Nouvelle Justine can perch so expectantly near the corner of Eighth Avenue. On a street that could run through Anywhere, U.S.A., you might as well be able to order a spanking for twenty dollars along with your fettuccine alfredo. Calling itself an "S & M café," La Nouvelle Justine offers food, drink, and innocuous, open-air adventures in domination, submission, and exhibition. The wait staff wear leather, netting, and ingeniously placed rings; they'll take your order from the specialty menu— twenty dollars for a spanking, a tickle session, or being fed like a baby in a bib and high chair—and smile gently as they help you pick your toppings: Would you like to be spanked with a paddle, or the hand? Tied to the beams in the center of the restaurant, or slung over Mistress's lap?

Despite the temptation of such titillating fare, I have come to La Nouvelle Justine merely for a drink—they have a two-for-one draft happy hour, and my friend Abby—Mistress Abby, to you—has provided me with a coupon for something fancy topped with an umbrella and fruit. Next to me at the bar is a couple who look to me like they might be in the wrong place; her shorts, sneakers, and carefully tanned legs, and his polo shirt and beard make me wonder if they have wandered in after a tough day of sightseeing. I don't know yet that Justine's is a highly favored tourist's destination, where office groups and bachelorette parties gather for lighthearted pinch-and-tickle. "What are you into?" The guy's voice is clear and earnest, as if we are all in a pediatrician's waiting room, and he's asking the weight of my newborn. "I'm into spanking," he offers helpfully. "I'm submissive."

I tell him—Nick is his name—that I'm into hair. "Do you wax for that?" I ask him, thinking maybe you get more bang for your buck if you wax your butt before the paddle hits. Nick nods thoughtfully, and I wonder if we're thinking the same thing. "So it hurts more?" He nods again, but more slowly this time. A second later, he understands that he's misunderstood. "Wax?" he says, "I thought you said, '*whacks.*'" One palm hits the other, very lightly; he's not a spanker himself. And no, he doesn't wax.

Nick's more concerned with the fact that he's losing so much on top; hair elsewhere doesn't bother him, and he hadn't previously considered the fact that ill-placed hair might dull the spanking sensation. He lives in Albany, New York, in fact, where I grew up, and he buys cases of generic Rogaine at the same discount warehouse from which my mother buys a month's worth of wine, paper towels, and toilet paper. He keeps it stored in the linen closet and uses it faithfully, twice a day. "I think it's working," he says eagerly, tipping his head toward me. Even the dull lights of the bar at La Nouvelle Justine glint off his barely covered scalp. He is pointing, asking me to judge. "I think it's starting to look normal, don't you?"

Of course, neither Nick's worries nor his hopes are simply the beer-soaked demons of a middle-aged submissive. In this, his presence at a darkened everyman's bar, where you can satisfy your deepest, most secret desires by ordering from a laminated card, is truly normal. Even before recorded history, Mexican cave painters rubbed their hopes and dreams for the future onto the dusky walls of caverns. They didn't pay much attention to detail, gesturing with line and color the gist of their desire for food, rain, and an adequate hunt, but one thing was immediately clear to the modern students who studied their work to understand their world: cavemen, too, went bald and submitted their scalps to public examination.

Perhaps the attentions of prehistoric peoples were of necessity directed elsewhere, perhaps no evidence to the contrary has survived, but it seems likely that it was left to civilization to devise remedies for the hair loss that the cave people must surely have considered more than an inconvenience in the hot sun and the cold winter. Though the Egyptians were a fastidious people, given to wholesale depilation and status-conferring wigs, in 4000 B.C.E. King Chata's mother recorded her recipe to make hair grow: grind together dogs' paws, dates, and asses' hooves; sauté in precious oil; and apply to the scalp. Hippocrates prescribed opium, wine, and "essence of rose," while the Romans tried bear fat and "viper's oil" from snakes trapped by the light of a full moon. Giovanni Batista della Porta, sixteenth-century author of a book on practical magic, advised his readers to pack their heads in "Man's dung burnt and anoynted with Honey," but those in need of immediate results were directed to try "burned barley bread, horse fat, and boiled river eel." And when Diane de Poitiers, balding mistress of Henry II of France, sought help from the illustrious Paracelsus, alchemist, physician, and student of the universe, he obliged with a vivid red liquid rumored to consist of blood from a birthing woman, a newborn, and the all-important "viper's wine."

Such potions are remarkable not because we've strayed so far from ancient wisdom—they almost certainly did not work—but rather because they are fraught with danger and mystery. They are imbued with a sacrificial quality that makes them desperate and heroic all at once—stalking snakes at the full moon, skimming blood from the birth canal, roasting human feces over an open flame, and then coating a bowed and hairless scalp. At the same time, their smoky, haunted aura reflects the enigmatic status of an unknown substance, neither skin nor tooth nor feather, a specific but inexplicable epithelial emanation. Hair lives as the human body lives and takes its nourishment from our blood, yet it lacks the capacity for sensory influence that joins our advanced opposable thumb with even the mute, light-fearing amoeba. It is of us, but feels no pain. Like restless spirits that belong neither to this world nor the next, hair has been invested with a totemic power by ancients and moderns alike. To keep from falling prey to "contagious magic," ancient warriors buried their hair trimmings, along with their saliva, nail clippings, and other bodily discards. In the hands of a malefactor, one's hair became one's weak and unprotected self.

The most glorious diamond in the world can bring queens to their knees and etch its name in glass, but it can't fight off even the humblest of thieves. Likewise, behind the shimmery curtain of its own mystery, hair remains a curiously vulnerable repository of power. It grows inexplicably and imperceptibly, with the legless movement of a snake; when it disappears, it takes with it all of the brawn it once bestowed. Indeed, in the mythical world baldness takes on its own mystique—the mystique of colossal, tragic defeat. Samson, whose strength knew no mortal equal, was shorn while his head lay prone on Delilah's knees. A chastened captive, his eyes gone and his spirit broken, when his scalp sprouted stubble he could only muster the strength to kill himself and the Philistines gathered to mock him. Taking their cue, no doubt, from Samson's fate, the colonial Dutch authorities in Amboyna realized early in their tenure that the hubris of native criminals resided in their hair: a quick visit from the barber could generally induce confession when all other tortures failed. Medieval European witch hunters had already learned a similar lesson. Imagining that the spirit consorts of their prey hid themselves in the witches' hair, they shaved many of their suspects clean. Most witches confessed soon after their forced depilation.

Satan himself, preaching in North Berwick, England, was supposed to have reassured his followers that they would be able to withstand anything, "so lang as their hair wes on."

Unfortunately, not even Satan could tell them how best to keep it; even devilish prescriptions failed those fated for baldness, whether the cause was political or genetic. Indeed, our modern medical remedies are not unlike their spooky counterparts from the past—elusive promise tinged with a hint of danger. Back-page ads still promise hair growth from herbal extracts, human placenta, and urea. Snake oil lost its reputation in the nineteenth century, so now we use biotin and other "hair nutrients"—wild bee honey, coltsfoot and onion juice, polysorbate 20, jojoba oil, and African Shea butter. Even Propecia and Rogaine, America's only FDA-approved hair-regrowth medications, share that appeal: their spokesmen wear baseball caps and smile their fears into the camera, but their ads also feature trick mirrors that project a baldheaded future for the perfectly hairy protagonist, and warnings worthy of the most ominous chain letter. Statistics show that approximately twenty-six percent of men between eighteen and forty-nine showed "moderate to dense" regrowth, and thirty-three percent showed "minimal regrowth" after four months of using a two-percent solution of Rogaine.

Most agree that Rogaine's biggest successes are in loss prevention, and Rogaine users humbly accept the rules: if you stop taking it, you'll lose all that you gained and, eventually, all the rest, too. Propecia statistics are as yet inconclusive—FDA approval was only recently given—though they don't promise to be wildly different from Rogaine's. Rogaine might make your scalp itch and swell, but Propecia wives beware: Propecia is not approved for use by women, and you shouldn't even handle your husband's pills if you are pregnant. While the side effects of Propecia are supposed to be minimal, they might include loss of libido and decreased semen volume. Wasn't there a note on the poison apple addressed directly to Snow White? I think it said, "Eat Me."

If the magical story of hair regrowth is a fairy tale, Don Hartman has stopped believing. He was in a Minoxidil study in the early 1980s and a Propecia study in the early 1990s, but neither medication provided the miracle he'd been looking for ever since he noticed his temples starting to deepen. Ever since, he'd had to admit to himself that thickening gels and special shampoos weren't going to keep his hair from falling out—he was going bald.

The thing is, Don has hair—not a lot of it, but enough to style and comb back, enough for him to run his hand through and, as it stands on end and flops over, remind himself that he needs a hair cut. He worries about it, he says, but it's not as important to him as it was in his twenties, when he first started to lose it and he thought to himself, Well, this is it. In fact, when we first sit down in a cocktail lounge at the midtown Manhattan Marriott, Don laughs self-consciously, because this isn't that big a deal to him— he's not sure why he even answered my ad. He's an actor, and instead of introducing himself with the usual small talk—hometown, brothers, sisters, mom, and dad—he hands me his portfolio and resumé: dark three-quarter shots, Don in a black turtleneck, almost Warren Beatty. He's been on *Matlock* and *Law and Order*. A Libra, just turned forty-five, Don knows exactly what I'm going to say before I say it. "Yeah," he says smiling with his hand up, "People guess me five to ten years younger."

It's early afternoon, not late enough for the blind dates that gather here on weeknights, nursing fancy drinks across low tables, and we've missed most of the tourists, who've already had their lunch and gone back out into the wan October sun. So Don and I are nearly alone in this piano bar, where the piano music is piped in for now, and he's certainly upbeat. He's been in New York a year and a half, and though he sometimes wishes he'd come north eight years earlier—he began his career in North Carolina, ten years ago—people say he's doing really well. He had lined up a waiter part in a movie called *Three Penny America*, but lost it when the producer and the casting agent who hired him had a falling out. So far, though, he's had several other promising moments: three lines as a plane passenger on *As the World Turns*, and though he didn't speak in his part as a juror on *Law and Order*, the camera focused on his reaction in a crucial moment. He was actually *the* jury. "It's hard to get through doors," he says, flagging momentarily. "There are so many actors . . . so many actors without representation." An agent, he thinks, would really speed things along. But for now, Don is determined, his Southern accent just noticeable enough to make him sound more cheerful, probably, than he really is. "I expect to be getting a phone call. Soon."

Still, he worries that "the hair thing"—he won't say anything more specific than that—limits his castability, especially for soap operas. "To me, bald is not beautiful." That's why he offered himself for the Rogaine and Propecia studies, and that's why, despite his misgivings and financial worries, he's still looking for a solution. Rogaine didn't really help, and since Minoxidil was originally a blood pressure medication, the prospects of a long-term commitment made him worry—"Is this going to lower my blood pressure too much?" It was the same with Propecia: though it was a blind study, Don was pretty sure his pill was the real thing, not a placebo, and that it was keeping his hair from falling out. The doctors even told him he was getting regrowth, and asked him to stay in the study. But he started getting concerned about side effects and the long term; would this affect his sex life eventually? And for iffy solutions, Rogaine and Propecia are quite expensive—thirty to fifty dollars a month. Even now, a friend swears that a product called Foladerm is making his hair grow back, and Don is ready to agree, but he doesn't have an extra fifty dollars.

"If I were a wealthy guy," he says, "I'd have already had transplants." A plastic surgeon once told him that he was exactly the type of patient he needed, and Don is sorry that ten to twenty thousand dollars is beyond his meager budget. He auditioned, once, for a Hair Club for Men commercial, but that was as an actor, not really as a prospective client. A hair replacement system—what we used to call a toupee—is not something he considers an option. Anyway, he didn't get the part. "I was lying—there was no way I'd wear that." He shrugs, shuddering just a little. "Maybe they picked up on that." He pauses, thinking about the possibility of wearing "a rug." "It would take a hell of a salesperson to sell me a system. Women wear wigs. Men don't."

The afternoon is wearing on, and Don has lost his original cheer. He's settled into the comfortable chair and into the lines on his face, and he's wondering if a receding hairline is going to keep him from being the actor he knows he could be; if maybe he'd made his move earlier, he'd have had more hair and a better chance. "If it takes me five years, I'm gonna be—oh my God—*fifty*." He's honestly surprised by the math. "I think, 'What if you don't make it as actor? What have you got?' If I give it up today, I've put so frigging much into this, I've got . . . absolutely nothing."

Don's hair has become not just a metaphor for his lost dream-world self, but also for his life as a whole. In the false dark of this piano bar, it seems thin, *receding*. What he wants is security. "Yeah," he says slowly, "more security. To have a little more in the bank. To be able to go to the doctor, or the dentist." *To get hair transplants.* He'd like to move out of the East Village, maybe to an apartment on Riverside Drive, or a loft in SoHo. "There are a lot of freaks [in the East Village]. I certainly don't feel like I fit in. It's a little bit dirty. I'd like to have an elevator building . . ." His voice trails off and he smiles, a bit self-conscious. He realizes, suddenly, that he's having an intimate conversation with a stranger, and again anticipates what he thinks I must be thinking. "I don't really have a lot of friends." This is his explanation for the conversation we've been having, as well as his final plaint. "That takes time, I guess." He and his partner, who sells suits on commission at Macy's, went to a party in Brooklyn last weekend, and already it's part of the past that by its very nature is irrecoverable. "That was nice—getting out," he says wistfully.

The truth is, Don's worried about it all, everything elusive in his life: his hair, his career, his health benefits, and that West Side elevator he'd like to ride on his way to work. When he's talking about the hair, the hair he's lost and won't get back, I drift a little, and when I come back, for a moment I'm not sure where he is, which part of his life he's mourning, powerless. "There's a part of me that wishes it really didn't matter," he says. "But the bottom line is that it does. I don't know how to make it not matter."

Eunuchs are not subject to gout; nor do they go bald.

—Hippocrates

Having conquered from sea to shining sea hindered only slightly by self-doubt and conscience, turn-of-the-century Americans were a uniquely confident bunch when it came to questions of cause and effect. Though social, political, and moral codes were in constant flux, few admitted their rapidly altering state, preferring instead the appearance, however false, of certitude. Hence, the sanctimonious yet scientific tone adopted for sociological discussions of such topics as racial types, poverty, and life in the tenements of New York City; and hence, too, the absolute surety of those who turned their attention to the hairless pates of modern society.

Like syphilis, hair loss was considered by many to be both a medical and a social concern. Ignoring the necessity of a particular array of microbes, social thinkers of the era considered syphilis—a stand-in for venereal disease in general—the natural result of a dissolute, dissipated lifestyle. As such, hair loss was the accepted effect of moral turpitude and a wanton neglect of polite standards, a physical punishment for a social crime. For those seeking a cause for the bald effect, there was no simply divined trail of evidence, no directly discernable smoking gun. Yet early theorists wrote with certainty anyway, sure that buried somewhere in the busy bustle of modern life, there was a reason for adult hair loss, especially in men. H. P. Truefitt, British cousin of American positivists, thought that modern man had made a Faustian bargain with the devil of scientific thinking. The devil's price, though, was not man's soul; it was his hair. Crowded with knowledge and churning with ideas, the modern man's cranial cavity had no room for the blood vessels needed to nourish thick, hearty follicles. "[T]he protracted and wearing exercise of thought," mused Truefitt, caused a "failure of nervous supply," then the "disappearance of fat from the cranial vault," and finally, baldness. In 1918, Richard W. Muller, M.D., turned Truefitt's theory upside down, flatly stating that it *was* fat that caused hair loss by promoting the spread of certain bacteria throughout the body. His recommendations: a diet, along with iron, quinine, and arsenic—thought to be a cure for syphilis, too.

A few years later, Charles Nessler, inventor of the permanent wave machine, published his theories in *The Story of Hair* (1928), a treatise meant to tell readers "the truth about human hair." Though his machines were used almost exclusively by women's salons, Nessler was deeply concerned with the care and preservation of men's hair, and devoted page after page to war metaphors and other masculine similes. Even a "battleship . . . is of relatively little importance to [the balding man]" wrote Nessler, "when he sees a vision of himself denuded of his hair, his scalp a scattering rink of venturesome flies." Nessler makes quick use of social science, associating hairiness with the primitive immigrants from the south and east of Europe, who exhibited their lusty, appetitive natures on their scalps and on their chests. Modern Anglo-Saxon men, in contrast, had weak scalps that mirrored their weak libidos and generally weak natures. American habits of cutting the hair of boys short only fed this trend toward baldness in its white men, since the scalp muscles never received the proper chance to develop through exercise; when middle age hit, they were flaccid and flabby, unable to hold onto the hair. By extension, flabby follicles implied lame reproduction statistics. In the Jewish community, warned Nessler, "hair production exceeds the non-Jewish races by at least five percent." Caucasian men, hairless and puny, were destined for "race suicide," unless they could breed at the frenzied pace set by the "bearded conquerors from across the ocean."

For Nessler, Truefitt, and Muller, there is an obvious connection between the challenges of modern manhood and what Nessler saw as a hair loss epidemic. (Indeed, Nessler warned women who bobbed their hair that they, too, might fall victim to scalp muscle atrophy.) To stay fit and firm when white collar professions required only minimal physical exertion, to harness as much "primitive" energy as they dared in order to stave off what Madison Grant called "the passing of the great race," must have seemed daunting tasks in a changing world. The early decades of the twentieth century spanned a period of upheaval in American gender roles: millions of immigrant men and women had recently arrived to soak up the lowest level of industrial jobs in urban centers; often, their ideas of masculine and feminine clashed with those of established citizens. During and after World War I, more and more women—young women especially—sought work outside their homes; the length of their skirts rose significantly, as did their expectations. In 1919, women were granted the right to vote. And in 1928, at the height of flapper visibility, in the crazy boom before the stock market crashed, Charles Nessler worried that lazy scalp muscles did not bode well for American manhood.

Nessler's conviction that baldness and virility are somehow crucially interconnected neatly reverses Hippocrates's ancient observation: eunuchs do not go bald. Aristotle, who was thinning himself, ruminated on the significance of this fact, adding a side note for the curious—eunuchs don't have chest hair either. But it wasn't until the 1950s that anyone was able to begin to uncover the link between castration and the longevity of head hair. Best known for his male pattern baldness classification system, Dr. James B. Hamilton also designed and conducted an experiment comparing hair loss in eunuchs and other men. With Hippocrates's remark as his starting point, he administered androgens (male hormones) to a group of eunuchs and watched their hair. Of course, the eunuchs given the hormones began to go bald, at the same rates and in the same patterns as their noncastrated male counterparts, slowly in their twenties, more quickly in their sixties. Clearly, Hippocrates was closer to the truth than Nessler. It is not the *absence* of masculinity that causes baldness, but rather, in a crude sense, its *presence*.

More than forty years later, the discussion retains the intricate, almost bellicose aura that marks the discourse of disease, technical nouns joined by warrior verbs. Follicles are choked, strangled, or suffocated when protective mechanisms and growth switches fail; the hairline pulls back, retreats, or marches aft. Reinforcements are essential, but hard to come by naturally; sometimes, it's necessary to purchase replacements—mercenary soldiers, they fill the ranks, but without the same dedication as native troops. And most disturbing, the enemy comes from within: 5-alpha reductase, a catalytic enzyme that converts the body's testosterone to 5-dihydrotestosterone, the form of the hormone that infiltrates the hair follicle and works to cut off its supply lines, so that, over time, healthy hair growth is impossible. If and when the hair regrows, following its natural cycle, it returns weaker and weaker each time, until eventually, it falls out permanently and the follicle dies. It's a military coup, of sorts, a stealthy but effective purge of front line troops effected from the inside out.

Of course, a perfectly run unit will not be as vulnerable as others. While there are no sure ways to prevent the onset of male pattern baldness, some trends have begun to emerge. Most importantly, a genetic predisposition must be present for 5DHT to work its deleterious magic; everyone has testosterone, 5-alpha reductase, and 5DHT in their systems, but not everyone succumbs to their assault. With the help of new radar, other sets of allies and enemies are slowly becoming visible. Nitric oxide, a substance that helps blood flow, may also promote hair growth. Superoxide, the release of which is possibly triggered by a toxic product of DHT, may react with nitric oxide to irritate, even poison, follicles; at the same time, it cues follicles to release their hold on the hairs already in place. Current thinking about nitric oxide and superoxide brings the blustery pronouncements of Muller and Truefitt back into play, since it seems there is a link between nitric oxide, heart disease, and follicle health: atherosclerosis certainly reduces production of nitric oxide, which may in turn limit its protection of hair follicles, making them more vulnerable to attacks of superoxide and DHT. Testosterone might be the tragic flaw of American manhood, both necessary and brutal, formative and destructive, but the ghost of Charles Nessler can't be banished altogether: nitric oxide is also thought to be instrumental in the work of erections.

It is probably the elemental nature of androgenetic alopecia—male pattern baldness, ostensibly caused by androgens, male hormones—that makes our medical remedies, the most prominent of which are Rogaine and Propecia, threatening and compelling all at once. Originally a blood pressure medication, Minoxidil (the active ingredient in Upjohn's Rogaine) caused an unexpected side effect in its original users: it caused them to grow hair where they had lost it. Probably because it is a vasodilator, Rogaine works to maintain the health of shrinking follicles, keeping them from suffocating under the influence of 5DHT. Though its efficacy as a tool for the restoration of hair is slowly being discounted, it appears to be an adequate intermediate measure, CPR for the follicles in full arrest. Merck's Propecia (finasteride) was originally developed as a prostate drug that reduces the production of 5-alpha-reductase, thus inhibiting the conversion of testosterone to 5DHT. Side effects, both potential and probable, seem to float right to the heart of the problem, linking Propecia at least in theory to more problematic androgen blockers: loss of libido, decreased semen volume, perhaps even gynecomastia (breast growth) for men. Many are hoping that Propecia and Rogaine can stall the inevitable until a true cure comes along, but no one is encouraging them to hold their breath. The *Wall Street Journal* reports that Merck chairman and chief executive officer Raymond

V. Gilmartin wears his hair in "what appears to be a classic side-to-side comb-over."

Vir pelosus, aut fortis, aut libidinosus
(*A hairy man is either libidinous or strong*)

—Latin proverb

Speculation about the physical causes of baldness builds on a long-standing association between hairiness and virility. The mistresses of the *Arabian Nights* framed it as a rhetorical question whose answer was understood implicitly and automatically. "Is there anything more ugly in the world," they asked, "than a man beardless and bald as an artichoke?" Havelock Ellis, the founder of the modern discourse on psychosexual dysfunction, asserted that the "vigour of the hairy system" is generally considered the "index of vigorous sexuality." He admitted that such an obvious assumption might at first seem unworthy of scientific discourse, but finally judged that in this case, "modern medical observations are at one with popular belief." It is not only natural, then, but also logical, that "strong eyebrows usually indicate a strong development of pubic hair."

Since this association is so deeply ingrained in our own popular imagination, which might have dismissed Havelock Ellis, but does not seem to have dismissed the Arabian mistresses, and since most remedies, from viper's oil to electric stimulation to DHT inhibitors have failed to recover lost hair, it is no wonder that when faced with external evidence of his own decline, a man would seek another means of replacing what he has lost. Caesar, fond of both his laurel crown and his brushed-forward 'do, since they worked together to camouflage his baldness, inspired a styling revolution for receding Romans. Wigs fashioned on Caesar's model did not have to finesse a part, and so had a better chance at verisimilitude. But others did not learn well enough from Caesar's example. Martial, the sharp-tongued satirist of the early empire, addressed an epigram in his sixth book to Phoebus, an optimistic Roman citizen who apparently eschewed wigs in favor of painted hair. "No need to call the barber for your head," Martial assured him. "A sponge can shave you better, Phoebus."

Although men's wigs remained fashionable through much of the Roman Empire, they were scarce in medieval England and France. It was not until the 1620s, when King Louis XIII went bald at age twenty-three, that wigs returned to the French courts, a device for concealment but also a badge of status. Despite the example of his father, Louis XIV resisted wigs as long as he could, growing his own hair long and curly until he was in his early thirties and his hair was too thin. After that, all of his courtiers sported huge white wigs, and Louis himself never showed his bare scalp to anyone except his loyal barber, Binette. At bedtime, he would pass his wig through the bed curtains to a waiting valet, and upon his waking in the morning, it would be passed back the same way. By the time Charles II took the fashion for wigs back to England with him in 1660, the revival was in full swing. For the next hundred years, wigs were so integral a part of social status in the Atlantic world that no one, tradesman, gentleman, or slave, need have worried too strenuously over impending baldness. Even in New England, where pride was a grave sin against social justice and the Reverend Increase Mather identified wigs as "horrid bushes of vanity," clergy and commoner alike were known to indulge. Indeed, Increase's son, Cotton, a right-ready judge of witches and other malevolent beasts, wore his wig often—but hopefully without pride.

Perhaps because wigs had become so readily identified with fashionable accoutrements in general, perhaps because the styles were often so large and elaborate, and the colors so improbable, eighteenth-century wearers took few pains to disguise their headgear. It was normal for wearers to lift their wigs for venting and scratching, even to remove the entire piece for a fight or a race (hence the expression "keep your hair on," a plea to the wearer not to get upset enough to warrant removing the wig). Though the wigs themselves were often controversial, mainly for religious reasons, their wig-ness was not.

But the young republic was not as comfortable with fancy and fashion as the eighteenth century had been, and by the middle of the nineteenth century, America had rejected the wig and its attitude of easy disguise for men. Urban wig sellers began promising a "gentlemen's invisible peruke," often made with a fine "hair lace cap," woven from human hair, that would allow the skin of the scalp to show through realistically. Some even used two layers of lace at the base of the part, so that individually knotted hairs could be drawn through the mesh of the top layer to simulate growth. The Sears catalogue of 1906 boasted toupees that would "defy detection," and by the 1950s, when the toupee made a comeback and men under thirty-five were purchasing the "Ivy League" style in droves, Sears mailed prospectuses in unmarked white envelopes. Men were considered the embodiment of republican tradition, the keepers of standards of objectivity, right, and wrong; for them to indulge in the cosmetic tampering that occupied women was, at least on the surface, a denial of their nature. Women were opaque, cloudy; men were supposed to be perspicuous, immediately intelligible. If keeping your hair was important in twentieth-century America, keeping your secret when you replaced it was even more important.

And it still is. Today's replacement venues are, like their forebears, institutions of discretion, if not discernment. As the public has gotten wise to some of the idiosyncrasies of replacement techniques, the industry has worked quickly to conceal whatever was exposed. The toupee, a reminder of the origins of hair replacement in full-headed wigs (the forepiece of which was called, in the eighteenth century, a *toupee*) has given way to a sleeker, more descriptive and scientific moniker, "hair replacement system," or, within the ranks, the familiar and confident "system." Stories of windswept hairpieces chased by chagrined suitors have been banished by promises of hypoallergenic glue and superstrong double-sided tape. Superfine mesh and paper-thin polyurethane disappear against the skin of the scalp and cancel the need for the thick, overlush bush or the long, fringed flap that we have come to associate with bad "rugs." It is a meticulous, cautious business, tuned to nuances of perception because, in the end, replacing hair is about nothing but perceptions.

But unlike most of his peers in the hair replacement business, Elliott Nonas thinks that linguistic contortions are for sissies. To Elliott, "system" is ridiculously pretentious. He wears leather pants to work and doesn't care if you call it a toupee, or a wig, or a hairpiece. He's been in this business for thirty-one years, he's eighty-three years old, and he can't understand what all the fuss is about. "Just don't call it a rug," he warns. That's going too far.

As the name might suggest, the Penthouse for Hair Recovery resembles a no-frills men's club, the kind of place where you can smoke all you want and no one will bother you. There is no moose head over the couch, but there are magazines with naked women inside scattered next to the couch. Pasted to the front of *Penthouse*—no relation, says Elliott, though I can tell it's a good association—is a typed notice: "This magazine is the property of The Penthouse for Hair Recovery. Any man caught stealing it will be publicly emasculated. Ladies will be forgiven." This is a big place, with workrooms and coloring rooms and several private cubbies tucked in the back, where the shy or squeamish can close the door, but Elliott's presence can make it feel small. He is tall, lean, and quick and never in one place for very long; his voice booms from behind the door of a consultation room, where a sheepish Asian man has followed him with his hands clasped behind his back. He greets everyone and tells them how they look before they ask. Along the walls are framed ad posters, reminders of Elliott's past. One is a stark picture of a black comb, several sad strands of hair caught in its teeth. Across the bottom is a simple question I hear in Elliott's gravelly voice: "Tired of combing your memories?"

Like most people in this business, Elliott began as a client—a "wearer," as they say, a "wearer" of hair—so he understands the practical and psychological urgency of hair replacement, the necessary depth of the illusion. The hair must not only seem real, it must be treated in all respects as if it were real; the point is not just to look as if you have hair, but to behave as if you have hair. You must be able, it seems, to fool yourself once in a while. Most people eat, sleep, and shower with their systems, styling their hair every morning with brushes and blow-dryers. They return to the Penthouse every few weeks to have them "re-bonded," and perhaps to have additional hair added, since hair replacement systems even shed realistically. With the old systems, swimming was impossible, because when the hair was wet it exposed the cap underneath, and, according to one former wearer, "looked like a drowned rat." But Elliott and his peers swear that the new fine mesh and polyurethane caps look just like skin, even when the hair is wet. Still, certain precautions must be taken. To keep his dates from touching his head and feeling the cap of his system instead of his hair, he used to warn them sternly early on. "Don't touch my head," he'd say, "I still have shrapnel from the war." Now, when he's talking to his bewildered young clients, he encourages them to embellish creatively. "You can make up a story," he urges. "But if you say, 'Don't ask me why—just don't touch my hair,' then that's all she wants to do! It seems to me, if you're in bed with a girl, she probably has other things to touch."

Elliott publishes a newsletter for his clients, *The Penthouse Papers*, in which he sets the tone for the business: masculine, humorous, cajoling. It is part stand-up shtick, part locker room pep talk. A rebel yell for the hair wearers. In short, pithy bursts, he demands to know why people make fun of baldness, and then boo and hiss at the prosthesis that corrects it. Who makes fun of wooden legs and glass eyes? What about dentures and breast implants? He ruminates on the popularity of the misguided comb-over, what he calls the "immigrant hairstyle" because it "comes from over there," and chides white men for thinking they can get away with shaving their heads when their hair starts to go. They think they look like Michael Jordan, he crows, but they don't! A sign in his office seems to sum up his ethos, the image he cultivates as a charm against the subtle implications of hair loss and, by extension, hair replacement: "Wise men go gray," the sign admits, but "rascals grow bald." It doesn't matter that most of Elliott's customers are not as bold or brave as he is, because for the few hours they spend each month in the Penthouse, where girly magazines remind them of their essential manly nature, and beautiful women touch their heads and make them whole, they can breathe the smoky aura of Elliott's pride. On their way out they poke around to look for him; they want a clap on the back before they go out onto the field.

It makes perfect sense, then, that Elliott's top of the line system would be called Virtual Reality. It is a name that calls on technological innovation, the wily ingenuity of machines that can successfully mimic something as rare as reality. It celebrates the trick of the clever system and, at the same time, thumbs its nose at reality because, really, there's nothing wrong with being nearly real, so like the real that it is, indeed, *virtually* real. Lace caps have been around forever, Elliott tells me, but the lace that is used for the Virtual Reality system is a fairly recent innovation, a "welded lace" that is strong enough to be kept on for sleeping, showering, and styling. It is sturdier, more transparent, and comes in eight shades so that Elliott can match the lace perfectly with the tone of your scalp. The lace at the front of the cap, which creates the missing hairline, is even finer than the rest, and because it is also more delicate, each Virtual Reality system comes with a set of extra fronts, which a client will have changed every five to eight months. Elliott beams when he talks about this system, which is virtually real, but also virtually undetectable.

"What do you think of mine?" he asks, pointing to the top of his head, where his white-gray hair seems to be thinning. For a long moment I am stuck, mouth open, brows furrowed. I have only just arrived, and my eyes have not yet adjusted to the light of Elliott's virtual world; I had thought that the hair on his head was really growing there—it was thin, but valiant, and arrayed in the deep V of men who are going to recede slowly for a long, long time. But when Elliott comes closer to show me the tiny knots that join the hair to the welded lace cap, a cap no bigger than my outstretched palm and light as paper, I adjust my focus until I can see a tiny piece of the virtual scalp, right in front, the unglued edge of a postage stamp.

Steve, who is twenty-eight and asks that I use his brother's name for this book, has had a system for ten years, ever since his hair first began to thin and he'd gone immediately to Bioexcell, another replacement company. That first piece wasn't dramatic or anything. "I had hair," he says, "but I was thinning and I couldn't take it." Ten years ago, there weren't very many other options, and Steve was fairly pleased with the results. "I wanted hair, and I didn't care how I got it." He shrugs. Now he's an expert in all the nuances, the hidden complications, that Bioexcell, like many companies, failed to mention on his first visit: the oxidation that changes the color of the piece if you spend too long in the sun, how the system itself loses hair and the cost involved in replacing it. "It falls out, like yours," he tells me, pleased to share his education. "But yours grows back." A contractor who admits that he "abuses" his systems, sweating, showering, blow-drying, and styling, Steve is not a good candidate for Elliott's delicate Virtual Reality. Steve's system is built on a heavier mesh base, and bonded with Be-Sure, an adhesive.

It is almost two, and Steve will be spending the rest of the afternoon at the Penthouse because his system needs ventilating—i.e., additional hair—and only after the hair has been added can Nancy, his stylist, rebond it. In the meantime, he sits at the long table in the back with Nancy, smoking and talking. She's been his stylist "forever"—when she came to work for Elliott, Steve followed her. They know the names of each other's families, and Nancy plays older sister to Steve's younger brother. He tells her she doesn't look her age—forty-one—and she tells him he should hold out for a nice girl who will appreciate him. He's glad to think about how long he's known her, to remind himself that she's there. "She's got a system, too," he tells me loudly, and she rolls her eyes. Her hair is long and layered, with bangs in the front; I can't tell if Steve was joking, exaggerating their bond, or not.

After a half hour or so, he orders a chicken sandwich and tries to get me to eat half. "Come on," he says when I decline, "what have you eaten for lunch?" Casually, between jokes with Nancy, he finishes his food. These are the only times that he is ever without his system, these the only people

besides himself who have ever seen the bald scalp underneath the thick auburn hair of his system, and he seems
relieved that there is one place, at least, where he doesn't have
to wonder if everyone's wondering what's up with his hair.

When it's time to start the gluing process, Nancy rests
Steve's system on his head and draws around it, through
his hair, with a soft black pencil. Then she uses a basting
brush to paint a band of glue just inside the black outline,
all around Steve's head, from forehead to crown and
back. The glue must be almost dry, tacky, before Nancy
can replace Steve's system, rolling it down from his forehead, stretching it every centimeter or so, so there are no
lumps or loose spots. So Steve has another wait, at least an
hour.

He's definitely more confident now than he would be if he
hadn't decided to replace what he's lost, but the double
vision of "virtual reality" can be straining sometimes. "You
still have that thing inside you that says, 'It's not my hair.' "
He laughs, thinking he sounds too picky, or deep. "But I got
a complex, you know? I'm always looking at my hair. I wonder if someone's looking at my hair, if they're gonna notice."
Hair, after all, is not like clothes; it's not like someone noticing your Levi's label. "Your hair *is* you—it's not something
you can buy—" He stops himself and laughs again. "Well, it
is now, but . . ." What he means is that it's not supposed to be.

Steve was married once, and engaged another time, but
lately he's just been going out with his buddies, to clubs like
Spy in Manhattan. He's sure that the reason girls are coming on to him lately is because his hair looks so great; if he
were out without his system, his bald dome would be the

only thing they'd see—no one would talk to him then. His first girlfriend went with him when he bought his first system, ten years ago, but after that, she never saw him without it. She said it really didn't matter to her either way, she liked him whether his hair was thin or thick, but he still doesn't believe it. Women say that all the time, but he thinks it must be one of those lies that they tell to spare men's egos. Another is that ring size doesn't matter. When he gave his former fiancée a diamond smaller than she wanted, she thanked him and said, "It's okay for now."

Steve shakes his head, because he feels that it's unfair, and still doesn't see how to get around it. There seems to be a connection between ring size and hair, but what can it be? He usually tells his girlfriends about his system, because "after about a month, they start looking at my hair, not at my eyes." He attributes this shift in focus from the eyes to the hairline to a sixth sense they have, but Elliott doesn't. From across the room he shouts at Steve, "It's because you wear it too low!" Elliott points to the black pencil mark on Steve's brow, and shakes his finger. "You have to move it up at least an inch!" Steve wants to know what I think—if I think his hairline is too low, and if I truly mind if a guy is losing his hair. We've reached a quick intimacy here, in this smoky room; I have now become one of the few people privy to his baldness. I can tell he thinks that maybe journalists believe more in the truth than other women. When I hesitate, he jumps right in. "I think you want a guy with lots of hair, don't you?"

Nancy has been following our conversation with a patient

smile. She's assumed long-term responsibility for Steve's security, and wants to put this ring question to bed once and for all. She turns to me, but her question is purely rhetorical. "Would you rather have a nice ring and be eating onions and bread at home? Or a T-bone steak and a smaller ring?" Hair might be important, she's saying, but food is essential.

In one of the back rooms, with the help of Paula, a long-haired Russian woman who also wears leather pants, Elliott is adjusting a new system his distributor convinced him to try. It is made with a wafer-thin polyurethane base that is supposed to be gas-permeable, and is meant to be worn just like the mesh ones, bonded on for four or five weeks at a time. Skeptical, but game, Elliott is trying it on himself first. He's not sure about the safety of polyurethane for long-term use; what happens to sweat and bacteria? This test is only the first step in his experiments, though, because he swears his own scalp doesn't sweat. "I don't drink water," he explains, "I only drink booze."

Paula removes Elliott's own system, which is secured with tape since Elliott doesn't sweat, and for a moment, Elliott is bald, a fringe of short white hair lacing the back and sides of his head. "This isn't me," he says, meeting my eyes in the mirror. "This is my father." While she cleans off his scalp and gets the new system ready, Elliott must sit and look at himself, hairless, in the mirror. His voice a little smaller than I've heard it before, he calls to Paula, "If I ever get Alzheimer's, you have to promise me you'll make sure I'm wearing my hair when I go out." Absently, Paula reassures him, but it doesn't work and suddenly he's gone from

Alzheimer's to death. He wants her to see to it that he is cremated. Now, Paula is paying attention. She roles the new system firmly onto Elliott's head, and suddenly, he has a head full of singular, flat gray curls. "Elliott," she says sternly, her accent only slowing her a little, "you're a Jewish man. If you get *cremated*, you're going straight to hell." Elliott ignores her and admires the curls even as she snips and they disappear. Using scissors with notched blades, like a comb, she blends the edges of the system with his own hair; then with water and a little gel she slicks the top back to show his forehead. He's calm again and death is a long way off. "I look very Roman," he says to me in the mirror.

Steve's system is back in place, too, and he's styling it himself like he always does. It is thick and spiky and maybe, like Elliott says, it comes down too low on his forehead. He's pleased, but wonders if maybe Elliott's right, maybe he's trying too hard, giving himself too much. "All I want is thin hair," he says, meaning, if it was all his own, he wouldn't mind it being thin. Twice, he's dreamed that he did have hair, that these past ten years were just an anxious nightmare. Both times, he woke up thinking it was true, and had to look in the mirror to remind himself it wasn't. Nancy stands behind him and shakes her head in sympathy. She speaks to his reflection in the mirror. "My dream is that I touch you guys like this"—she lays both hands on his head, a healing gesture—"and all the hair grows out." Her fingers tap his head and sprinkle away like glitter.

Hair

Indeed, can a bald headed woman successfully arouse emotions of love?

—Charles Nessler, *The Story of Hair*

A few years ago I was in the waiting room at my general practitioner's office, along with everyone else who had been taken by surprise by that year's flu. Aching and feverish, I was paying little attention to what was going on around me, sure only that I would hear the familiar ring of my own name when it was time to see the doctor. These were the early days of managed care, before we all got savvy about fax machines, and several people who had not yet been visited by the flu were defying germ probabilities and picking up referrals. Through the haze of my fever I remember a slight woman in pink sweatpants, a red parka, and a black beret, leaning as best she could through the receptionist's window. She came for her referral, she said, to a doctor what's-his-name. The receptionist must have had to fill in the cause, or her complaint, on the form because then I could hear the woman mumble. The receptionist cupped her ear. "What?" she asked.

"Female pattern baldness," the woman said.

"Excuse me?" The receptionist was, and still is, an awfully nice woman; she just couldn't hear her.

"Female pattern baldness," she said, a little louder this time, and a little more slowly.

"I'm sorry," said the receptionist, meaning it. She stood to get closer. "One more time."

"Female pattern baldness!" The woman yelled this shrilly, her voice skidding through the waiting room. In another second, she had gathered her referral and was gone.

∞

Waiting room humiliations aside, history has, in some sense, been kind to balding women. By generally offering, at least, the refuge of cosmetic artifice, it has made it possible for the record to reflect generations of stylistic whimsy, rather than centuries of anguished hair loss. From the earliest days of civilization, we have evidence of elaborate wigs and headdresses. Ancient Egyptian women wore wigs made of gold; eighteenth-century gentlewomen stretched hair over wire frames and adorned the structures with flags, boats, and bird nests. For much of our own century, it was improper and impolite for a middle class woman to venture outside without a covering of some sort.

At the same time, Judeo-Christian, and later Muslim, standards of modesty long required women's hair to be covered, since it was considered so personal an appendage, and thus, so seductive a revelation. Men's hair has long functioned as a symbol of virility, the quiescent possibility of conquest, and likewise women's hair has always been connected to women's sexuality, the difference being that this female sexuality is often construed as a danger to men: Medusa's snaky locks propelled enemies toward her eyes; Lorelei, mythical siren of the Rhine, untangled her golden tresses while she awaited unsuspecting sailors; and medieval Europeans shaved suspected witches because it was thought that the evil demons that guided them nested in their hair. Hence, a dualism that haunts us today: a simultaneous exaltation and demonization of female hair, an elevation that for centuries required that the vaunted treasure be hidden.

And yet, despite the services it offered cultures that required covers for female features, be they too lovely or too unlovely, cosmetic subterfuge has its own ambivalent history. During moments of military aggression, the Roman assembly banned makeup and hair dye, along with excessive displays of jewelry, lest women distract soldiers from the tasks at hand. Even in times of peace, writers like Martial mocked Roman women for their reliance on wigs: "The golden hair that Galla wears/Is hers—who would have thought it?/She swears 'tis hers and true she swears,/For I know where she bought it."

The issue, of course, was never simply one of conspicuous consumption, but generally one of deception. If marriage is chiefly an economic exchange, a transaction of acquisition for the new husband, it is only fair that he know exactly what he is purchasing. In 1770, the British parliament debated a bill that railed against women who used "scents, paints, cosmetic washes; artificial teeth, false hair, Spanish wool" or even "high-heeled shoes or bolstered hips" to "lure any of his Majesty's subjects" into matrimony. These women were considered witches and were to be punished accordingly. *Ladies Home Journal* published a letter in 1911 from an irate newlywed, chagrined by his wife's hair deception. "The step from the wearing of a lie to the acting of a lie is not a long one," he warned.

The result is an ambivalent record: an elaborate line of wigs and head coverings, stretching from the ancient world to modern times; a western cultural legacy haunted by snaky curls, raven tresses, and shorn witches; and a hair market that waxes and wanes, depending on the styles, but usually advertises on the back pages. The bottom line is that though fashion has always made it easier to hide, female hair problems have probably been around forever. The seven Sutherland sisters from upstate New York toured the country to display their floor-length hair, the longest in the world, supplementing their income with sales of their special formula Hair Grower and Scalp Cleaner—hope for those who weren't as fortunate. Madame C. J. Walker, the first black woman to become a millionaire in the United States, made her fortune with an implicit promise to straighten black curls, but her most popular product was the Wonderful Hair Grower.

The twentieth century has offered some opportunity for easy camouflage, but since the Afro wigs and bouffant falls fell into disuse (their brief 1990s revival was truly brief) and modesty no longer requires hats in daily life, the average thin-haired woman hasn't had many options. Some have had success with Rogaine—according to the *FDA Consumer*, twenty percent between the ages of eighteen and forty-five experienced moderate regrowth; forty percent experienced minimal regrowth—but many more haven't, and no Propecia-like drug is on the market yet for women. Over twenty million women suffer from androgenetic alopecia—female pattern baldness caused by the same hormones that cause male pattern baldness—but dialogue has been slow in starting. This is the kind of secret women have always been very, very good at keeping.

In her first year of graduate school, Anita Angelone began losing her hair for the second time in her life. The first doctor she consulted looked at the quarter-sized bald spot just behind her hairline, shook his head and shrugged his shoulders. "It's either gonna come back or it's not," he said. "And you know what I think? I think hair is overrated in Western culture." The second doctor provided a diagnosis, but no cure. "Alopecia areata," he said, meaning literally, baldness in a specific, contained, usually round spot, or spots—*area baldness.* He recommended a haircut at Barney's. The haircut didn't really help, but Anita figured she was finally on the right track. She went to the Gap and bought a green corduroy newsboy cap and wore it every day.

With an easy laugh and a lingering trace of Texas drawl, Anita seems confident and poised. She's spending this summer studying for her Ph.D. oral exams in Italian literature and culture, dividing her days between the gym and the library exactly the way she's supposed to be; to force herself to relax, she attends a swing-dance class where she's gotten good enough to wish she could be picky about partners, even if she hates to be mean and say no if someone asks. Her thick, wavy light brown hair is tousled and chin length, and it doesn't show even a hint of hair trauma, but both of her Italian-born parents are hairdressers and adolescent rebellion in their house was switching from Dad to Mom for a change in style. What's more, her mother has a thyroid problem, and as a result, her hair is thinning. When a bad car accident several years ago put Anita in a coma for two and a half weeks, and her hair started to fall out in clumps from the shock—the first time she lost her hair—this was what she pictured, the final pronouncement of genetic destiny. I'm gonna have hair like my mom's, she thought. Her radar's tuned; she's perceptive, even vigilant when it comes to hair. Anita is wired for hair trouble.

She also believes in a sort of hair karma, a universal balance that governs hair fortunes according to a reciprocal, almost religious logic that goes beyond the expectation of genetics. Mere chromosomes would counsel thyroid problems, not alopecia areata. Anita remembers that when her hair started to fall out, her then boyfriend was extremely comforting and supportive—he'd kiss her bald spot and declare it loved. But as her hair started to grow back, and her self-confidence returned, they started to grow apart. He dumped her for a friend of hers, a woman who had and still has "an incredibly fluffy part." Anita's still bothered by the betrayal, and by the image of her own envy. "I was incredibly jealous of that part," she says now, laughing even as her eyes narrow and she shakes her head. "I didn't realize all I had to do was blow it dry."

Her former roommate is part of the cycle, too, another piece in the karmic puzzle. This woman, a psychologist, had thick, curly black hair that seemed to Anita to be shedding constantly. "There were these tumbleweeds floating across the apartment," says Anita. Annoyed, she confronted her, hoping for a cleaner apartment. It was only later, though, when Anita's own problem surfaced, that her roommate confided the source of the tumbleweeds: she suffers from trichotillomania, an impulse disorder that makes people pull out their hair, strand by strand. She, too, was worried about hair loss—her hair was not growing back as fast as she was pulling it out, and she was noticing thin spots. "I felt like I got what I deserved," says Anita, only half-joking. Trying to reassure her, I tell her essayist Edward Hoagland's version of karmic reciprocity: one day, as a young boy, Hoagland teased a playmate about his stutter; soon after, Hoagland himself was stuttering, twice as bad as his friend. He still does. Anita nods absently, her thoughts lingering on the tense memory of two young women losing their hair in one apartment. "I'd hear the hair snap out," she says, "and I'd tell her to stop. She'd say, 'Thanks.'"

Alopecia areata is a still something of a mystery to researchers, but it seems to be an auto-immune disorder that causes the body's defenses to misidentify and then attack its own hair follicles. It's hard to guard against this kind of intruder, the kind that sneaks up from within, coming without warning to steal your most vulnerable asset, the one you expected to lose some day and can't protect. Anita's only defense is a storekeeper's vigilance: inventory. She combs her fingers through her hair in the shower, gathers what's come out, and sticks it to the tiled wall. Then, one by one, she counts what she's lost. "Today, I lost gobs of hair in the shower," she says, a little shaky. "And when I was blowing it dry, I lost gobs. There were too many to count. But I tell myself, it's not all from one place." Two years later, she's still waiting for it to happen again. The gym, she thinks, will save her. "As long as I do that. . . ." She makes a fist, pumps it. "As long as I keep myself strong in that way . . . I tell myself, 'As long as I keep working out, nothing bad will happen.'"

Before Elline Surianello lost count, she'd used 110 things today—the toilet, the sink, the shower. She's counting because she's a problem solver by nature, that's how she got into the hair replacement business, and because she thinks there must be an alternative to the frenzied pace she's been keeping since she started this nine years ago. A small woman with a booming voice, Elline keeps her shoulders back and her lips closed when she's not speaking. She began

Le Metric after searching avidly for a solution to her own hair problems and finding almost nothing in place for women—no treatments, no replacement alternatives, nothing but wigs and hats. At first only a training initiative for stylists in Buffalo, New York, in which she and her partner, Cliff, taught weaving techniques they developed on Elline, by May 1992, Le Metric had evolved into a full-scale New York hair replacement salon and Cliff had died of AIDS. Now Elline designs and creates hair replacement systems with the help of four ventilators, four stylists, and a three-person support staff. Last year, she moved Le Metric from a six-hundred-fifty-square-foot office to a twenty-five-hundred-square-foot office, and now she fields almost two hundred customer inquiries a month. Today, a busy pre-Christmas Saturday, the salon is bustling, the candy dish on the reception desk is full, a vanilla candle silently scents the air, and Elline is using a spare moment to think about having so little time to think. She sits for a second in the receptionist's chair and admits, "I don't remember my mother spending so much time saving time." Then she gets up to sweep the floor.

Elline's mother might not have devoted herself to her own energy conservation, but she did mull over her daughter's thin and thinning hair. When Elline was ten, she shaved it all off, promising her daughter that it would grow back thicker. "It didn't do shit," Elline says now, with a certain stoic distance and a flash of fatalistic humor. Early on, she accepted thin hair as her destiny, and "never really felt in a crisis about it." She had good clothes, makeup, a cute body, and wore her hair short through the seventies; it was only later, when the problem got significantly worse and her body began to settle into maturity that Elline felt she had to take action. In 1984, she took stock. "Your body changes; you're not real cute anymore. How do you go and do work when people are staring at your head?" To this day, Elline maintains that for women, hair replacement is as much a public, economic decision as anything else. "Women don't age as well as men do," she insists. If a balding man and a balding woman were walking down the street at the same time, Elline asks, "guess who's gonna get looked at?" She doesn't need to wait for an answer. Men worry about their hair for themselves and their egos; women know that it affects everything—their self-esteem, their sexuality, their performance at work.

Before she started Le Metric, Elline worked for Revlon as a makeup artist; she sold office equipment and other things people weren't sure they needed when she first walked in; after that, she worked for her family's construction business in Buffalo, helping to make and market concrete highway dividers. She has that raw, irresistible salesperson's energy that promises both empathy and aid. The difference is that now she's developed a product for a need she didn't create—it was already there, a gaping hole in the market and in the psyches of millions of women.

When Elline started there was nothing even for her to research, no avenues to investigate. She had to develop a product with no real market precedent and assemble the financial and technical support to produce it, starting from ground zero. Hair replacement systems were for men, and wigs were for women—there was nothing in-between. "Who do you call? Nobody. I couldn't even *steal* the information," she says emphatically. Raw materials were also an issue, since the international hair market is also extremely insular and competitive. "It's like the diamond business, you just gotta know. And really good hair is even more valuable than diamonds." This secret is hard won and fiercely protected. Elline smiles when asked, but won't say where or how she buys her hair, only admitting that "hair is very, very expensive." Someone—probably someone without the connections she has—might pay anywhere from one hundred sixty to three hundred dollars an ounce for good quality European hair. From a plastic bag she pulls a system she's designed and drapes it over her hand, shaking it so that the hair, blond and shimmery, shows off its highlights. Her smile is knowing, challenging. She buys good hair.

The phone behind the desk buzzes—it's someone who wants information, so Elline swivels her chair around to take the call. Her head bends and she is what she's supposed to be, empathetic and prescriptive, a comfort but also a kick in the pants. "I happen to wear hair all the time," she says. And then, "That doesn't work, girlfriend! That's why you're callin' me!" When Elline hangs up, she swings back around and shakes her head. "She hasn't even concluded yet there's no way to get hair back."

The open floor plan, manicure station, and shelves full of styling products make Le Metric seem like any other busy, upscale Manhattan salon. The fixtures are modern, the music is quiet—only the iron spools clamped to the counters signal any change from the ordinary. These hold the thread that Elline's stylists weave into a client's own hair, forming a narrow circular track. From a distance of a few feet, these tracks look like hair jewelry, headbands and tiaras, signs of royalty and status, not anchors for the mesh bases of hair replacement systems. Really, this is the genius of Elline's creation, keeping these women out of private cubbyholes, where their loss can fester like a secret shame, and making the accoutrements of the replacement system, the woven track, the netted mesh, someone else's hair, seem like the tools of an exotic adornment ritual, like an intricate henna design painted on the palm.

Marianna, who wore for a wig for fifteen years before discovering Elline, respects her system. She can keep it on for five to six weeks at a time, having it washed and set once a week at a shop in her neighborhood, returning to Elline's only to have her track tightened and her system reattached. A mesh cap that covers the top of her head and reaches only slightly to the sides, it is far lighter than any wig she owned; and yet, it is far more powerful, more realistic, and more transforming all at once. She had never felt like the wigs were hers—they were more like hats than hair. This system is a part of her.

Indeed, it is like the best parts of her turned out toward the world, allowing her to hide the rest. Beneath the system, Marianna is nearly bald over much of the top of her head, not because she's suffering, like Elline, from androgenetic alopecia, but because she pulls her hair out. She has trichotillomania, and though she's searched for ways to cure or at least curb her habit, this system is the only thing that's helped. She's tried Rogaine, but her follicles are too damaged; she doesn't expect too much of her hair to come back, even if she could allow it to. She's also tried Paxil—an antidepressant used to treat obsessive-compulsive disorders—but didn't feel like the results were worth the side effects.

When she was a teenager, her parents forbid her to pull her hair, urging her to sit on her hands and buying her mittens to still her fingers. Later, she tried psychotherapy and behavioral modification therapy. "It's basically—stop that, don't do that," she says, rolling her eyes at the impossibility of the obvious. "It's not like you wake up in the morning and say, 'Boy, I really wanna do that.'"

Her system and its needs are one of the few things that have penetrated the single-minded logic of her disorder. Sometimes, when she reaches to pull out her hair and feels the system, it shakes her out of her trance and helps her to put her hand down. More urgent is her worry about the integrity of the track, because without it she'll have to go back to a wig. If she pulls out too much, she knows soon she won't have enough to wind the thread around. To Marianna, these are challenges, though, obstacles that make life harder but no less enjoyable. She can't drive over bridges, either. "It stops me from going certain places," she admits, but it forces her to be creative as well, to find another route. She sees her hair loss as a similar problem. Pointing to her head, where the dark line of the track stands out against a nearly bald scalp, she says, "This is an incentive, to see what I can accomplish."

She had a client once, Elline tells me, who tried to jump out of Le Metric's office window when she saw herself with her system on for the first time. "If you have no hair and then suddenly, you have hair . . ." Elline's voice trails off. This woman was like a hunger artist suddenly gorging herself on chocolate cake—she choked on the luxury of her hair. "Her acknowledgment that that's how she walked around was too much." The woman returned an hour and a half later, calm, ready for her transformation. Over time, she lost weight, and gradually she got used to her new self. But Elline's still stunned by the story—the dramatic rush of this woman toward the window, and her own understanding; she saw immediately why the improved image in the mirror was so devastating.

Elline lifts the front of her system to prove her point, exposing her sparsely covered scalp. She means to show me the complicated construction of her system—a lace cap in front, with a series of crossed wefts in back; a lot of hair attached to a small area of mesh, it falls from the top of her head so that her improvised bun, held together with a pencil, shows her natural hairline in back—but it's also a moment of aggressive exposure, a chance for me to cry uncle and cede the floor. There's a lot of anger floating through here, she'd told me earlier, a lot of deep, pent-up emotion. She'd been discussing a couple of Long Island women who'd asked if she could design extensions for them; they wanted long hair but didn't have the patience to grow it. Money was no problem, they'd said, when she warned them that her hair is extremely expensive. In the end she'd refused and sent them away. "I don't do women who want fun hair," she said.

As Marianna gets ready to leave Le Metric, her system reattached, colored, and set, Elline steers her toward Rhonda, another hair-puller, who's been taking an herbal mixture she purchased in California to help curb her habit. The problem is, Rhonda doesn't remember what is in the capsules besides St. John's wort, though she swears it's working. She takes one in the morning, with her vitamins, and then another whenever she gets the urge to pull. They calm her down, she says, and quell the need. When she goes back to California, she promises Marianna, she'll find out exactly what this mixture is. Marianna, however, looks skeptical. She smiles at Rhonda and wishes her luck, but she doesn't have faith in remedies anymore—she has faith in her system.

Rhonda has been able to keep more of her hair than Marianna. She started pulling from a spot just to the left of her part, right at the top of her head, and then the urge spread a little to the side. If you look at her from the front, the bald area is not even visible. Because it is so contained, Rhonda is able to wear a small system, just big enough to cover the area and still blend well with the rest of her shoulder-length hair, and it is not attached with a track, just clips that comb into the hair she's got. She's only needed to wear a system since her late thirties, after a long relationship ended and her pulling urge got particularly intense, but she thinks that with these new capsules, she might not keep it too much longer. Though behind her Elline's frown shows that she knows better, Rhonda fixes optimistic blue eyes on mine and estimates that it will take two years, tops. Her discovery of St. John's wort coincided with "those changes" that necessitate hormone replacement, and she believes in her regimen and its power to restore whatever has been lost. The clips help keep her focused on her goal of quitting. "When it gets sewn into your head, you kind of give up," she says, without mentioning Marianna or anyone else she's encountered here at Le Metric. Ignoring Elline, Rhonda leans toward me and shrugs. "I seem to have some kind of faith that it will come back."

A clothing designer who just began her own company, Rhonda smiles with a quiet calm that might be confidence, or might even be forbearance. She's bewildered by this impulse of hers, but not overly concerned. She never considered herself an anxious person, but she knows she must be, somewhere inside of her. A quick shift in perspective, and pulling is a helpful mechanism that keeps other trouble at bay. Her bald spot is just a bull's eye or a voodoo talisman, "one prime spot where all of this anxiety is centered." It is a receptacle for otherwise harmful waste. Rhonda's been to therapy, but she never thought it was important to tell the therapist about this; she had enough emotional terrain to cover—her mother, her work, her other relationships. There was no need to discuss an impulse so natural and restorative. She skates over the bald spot and offers an axiom that raises as many questions as it answers. "When you look normal," she says, "you are normal."

This is important because sometimes, perception is everything—for Rhonda and for the enterprise of hair replacement. Sometimes, it only matters what the mirror says. Nearing fifty, Rhonda lives alone and has never been married; she has no children and no steady boyfriend. Over time, she's noticed that her friends, her colleagues, even random people she meets, greet childless, unmarried middle-aged women with pity and low expectations. The dinner invitations come a little less frequently as more of her friends marry, and people wonder, as Rhonda never does herself, what her reason is for getting up in the morning. Rhonda admits that her hair secret, kept from even her closest friends, is "another reason why I have to live alone," a reason to keep her own hotel room when she goes on vacation with friends, perhaps even a reason to shy away from romance altogether. Still, she won't give an inch to stereotypes, and she won't pity herself the way others seem to pity her. She looked at her college graduation picture recently, and she really thinks she looks the same, "except for a slight aging in my face." Wearing her system is "like having a face lift." It smoothes the surface and wards away the demons.

I walk outside with Rhonda, into the bright sun of an empty Saturday in midtown Manhattan. She's forgotten her hair already and is excited about an idea she has for my next book. "You should write about successful women who are approaching fifty and are alone," she urges. "It's a huge part of the population now." She promises me both readership and sales; I'm not sure if she's offering to be my subject. "Really, it's a great topic." But in the seconds it takes me to consider her proposal, Rhonda's already going the other way, her hands deep in her pockets, her pace slow but sure.

The obstacles in the way of restoring the hair are great, inasmuch as . . . we have to attempt the restoration of function in an organ which . . . is not only impaired in vitality, but has actually ceased to exist.

—H. P. Truefitt, 1863

In his counseling office on Long Island, Neil Henry keeps an old photograph of his first fourth-grade class, a smiling group of kids arrayed somewhat shyly around their young teacher. Talk with Neil about this picture, and he remembers how difficult that year was, his first year of teaching in East New York. He'd chosen that classroom over Vietnam, but in the middle of the year he considered becoming a fighter pilot after all—he had great eyesight, and these kids were much harder to handle than he'd expected. Eventually, though, he decided to stick it out with the kids—a good thing, he thinks. Look at this picture with Neil, though, and he's no longer interested in education, Vietnam, or his fond memories of those tough little kids. Now, he notices two things: the orange jacket he found in the incinerator room of his building ("This is my jacket now," he said), and his hair. "I had all of my hair then." He's not sure whether he's surprised or not, so he says it again. "I had all my hair!"

It was later, of course, when he was already married, that he started to notice the change. Badly placed mirrors and other reflective surfaces reminded him of what he worked hard at forgetting. "I tried to fool myself." He laughs now. "I'd hold my head a certain way—I *know* people can fool themselves." Before bar mitzvahs and weddings, though, his wife and kids would remind him, telling him he needed an extra-big yarmulke to cover his bald spot. The final straw was a vacation video, shot while he was swimming naked in the Rio Grande. He remembers watching the video and speaking to himself like the army drill sergeant he never had. "There is a fat elephant who is bald! I know looks are superficial, but they're not. . . . You're getting a hair transplant." Now, almost five years later, he's had a scalp reduction and a grand total of 1,087 hair grafts, which cost him, in the end, just a little more than a dollar per hair. In his files he keeps a card with the stats for each transplant session typed in columns. He was supposed to be finished two sessions ago, but he's seen results and is getting greedy. "Oh, you have hair?" he says to himself. "Guess what—it could be a little thicker." So far, he's spent $10,600.

∞

Moving hair, follicles and all, from the back of the head, where it generally continues to grow in abundance even after the onset of androgenetic alopecia, to the top and front of the head, where it has ceased to grow, is generally considered the end of the line in hair recovery. It is the expensive, painful, bloody process you undergo after you give up on Rogaine and nearly-real replacement systems, and finally decide your life is a wash unless you get some hair up there—in other words, when you're a fat, bald elephant and you need hair transplants. Like fertility treatments, this is a last-ditch effort to preserve and extend genetic material, to "sew" your own seed, so to speak, with the help of modern medicine. Hair transplants reject plastics for plasticity, building on the belief that the surface of the body can be morphed and stretched into something better and more beautiful than it already is. It is surgery for an elastic but literal age: it doesn't matter where the hair comes from, or how it gets there, as long as it is embedded in the scalp and sprouts from skin.

Gary Hitzig, the surgeon who performed Neil's transplants, practices what he preaches. Like many of his clients, he furiously sought other remedies for his hair loss, paying fantastic sums for cow urine ointments and replacement systems. He knows all the tricks, trials, and traumas of the hair replacement racket and has his own version of every apocryphal hair replacement tale. To hide the fact that most of his hair was a carefully camouflaged system, he asked his dates to please not touch his head, because it was still very sensitive from an accident in his Volkswagen Beetle where his head had gone through the windshield. Once, a violent gust of wind stole his system while he was walking with a date on York Avenue. He chased it, caught it, and kept on running all the way to his car; he never spoke to his date again. Though he began his own hair transplants twenty-five years ago, long before the advent of Rogaine and Propecia, he's pretty sure these drugs wouldn't have changed anything for him, as they don't for most of his patients, except maybe to postpone the inevitable. Nor is he convinced that Propecia, for instance, is safe enough for long-term use. "Fen-Phen was safe and effective until Fen-Phen wasn't safe and effective," he reminds me. Blocking DHT might be a dangerous thing, especially for men hoping to father children. The world of hair replacement turns some received medical wisdom upside down, it seems, making drugs more dangerous than surgery.

Gary Hitzig's a good-looking guy, a successful surgeon who skis in Aspen with his wife and steers the conversation to his twins, Carly and Ben, whenever he possibly can. He says, for instance, that the latest transplant techniques make the hair look much more natural when it's wet, so he doesn't have to worry when he's swimming with his kids. But for all his confidence and poise, he hasn't fully exorcised the ghost of that awkward young guy who lost his toupee on a date with a girl. Though his first wife knew he'd had transplants, he never allowed her to see him with wet hair, since that was when the plugs were visible. When I express surprise, *he* looks surprised, shrugs, then looks away. "You don't want to come out and look like an eyesore to people," he says. This is why he's so thrilled with his hair now, having undergone transplants with the benefits of all the latest technologies. This is probably also why he loves his work—it's a healing endeavor for himself as well as his patients, repairing the wounds of the geek he used to be.

Of course, it helps that hair transplant techniques combine the latest technological innovations in the service of a good old-fashioned ideology of conquest, the *X-Files* meets John Wayne on the set of *Bonanza*. The entire enterprise is predicated on the principle of "donor dominance," the idea that the donor hair from the back of the head, once implanted, will retain its old growth patterns and not succumb to the weaknesses of the hair it is succeeding. Tiny round-bladed scalpels cut lines of donor follicles from the back of the head, and new linear graft cutters, invented by Dr. Hitzig himself, slice both the new hair and the slits in the scalp to be small, intact, and exactly the same size. To speed the healing of the graft sites, Dr. Hitzig employs an infrared coagulator, which uses defocused infrared light to cauterize surface wounds. When he shows me the linear graft cutter he designed, he handles it respectfully, lovingly, almost like a pen he could use to carve his name in your scalp. He smiles and tells me just how sharp this baby is: "If I dropped this," he says, "it would slice right through your foot."

This is the masculine end of the plastic surgery profession we normally associate with breast implants and tummy tucks, and it has a cowboy-and-Indian feel to it that is hard to ignore. Although the modern technology really got its impetus from industrial scalping accidents, an almost exclusively female phenomenon involving long hair and the omnivorous "revolving shafts" of early factories, there remains a trace of frontier danger. J. S. Davis, a scalp-grafting pioneer from Johns Hopkins, published a graphic treatise on his work in

1917 entitled, simply, "Scalping Accidents," which evokes this ranger's resourcefulness with pictures of a leather punch and a button-holer he used to section grafts from strips of skin. Fifty-three of the fifty-four cases he mentions belong to women, several of whom were "raised to the ceiling and dropped to the floor" by the machines that grabbed their hair and, in a number of cases, ripped off their eyebrows and ears as well. But one man overshadows all fifty-three of those women, though his entry is brief and laconic: he lost his scalp to the Indians in Nebraska and survived to undergo scalp grafts. They were, Davis assures us, successful.

Neil Henry tells his story in a way that pays homage to the comics of the 1930s, when the cowboys became G-men and the bad guys went out with a "kapow!" In his tale, he's the average guy who ignores his wife's constant patter of dissent, and slips into a phone booth to change into a superhero with shiny dark hair. Neil's also a Long Island therapist who might as well moonlight as a stand-up comedian, since men's insecurities are incredibly funny these days. "My wife, as usual, thought I was nuts," he remembers. But once he made up his mind, he was determined. It was 1994, and he was still driving an '82 Corolla his parents bought him so he could get to work on time. He thought, "I could get a new car, or I could have hair on my head. No contest. I'm workin', I'm payin' my bills, and I wanna have some hair on my head!" He had the transplants, kept the car, and now his wife is his ex-wife. "I like when people say, 'Oh your hair looks nice,' " he explains, "as opposed to 'You have a bald head and we won't say anything about it.' "

Not once has he been embarrassed about his decision. When he returned home after the first transplant, his head wrapped in bandages, he hailed his neighbors. They were horrified, but he was elated. "Boy, do I feel good," he told them, "I just got hair transplants!" Now he jokes that he even tells some of his patients, when he thinks it will help their body image problems. "I know we're talkin' about how you're gonna commit suicide," he says to the imaginary patient on his couch, "but, notice anything different about me?" He points to his head and grins. His only worry now is that his parents will read this book and discover that he spent so much money on his hair. "No really," he insists when I laugh. "If there's a rubber band in the middle of Sunrise Highway, my mother will stop to pick it up." I must look skeptical, because he touches my arm, trying to push me to see he's serious. "I'm only saying this because it's true—it really happened."

There's a giddiness to all these guys, these men who've beaten the bad guys and found a way to keep their hair. They tell their tales with end-of-the-day bravado, willing to reveal how bad it was in order to show off how good it is. I mention this to Hitzig, my surprise at how urgent the secrets used to be and how easily they are shared now. He smiles, maybe because he thinks I'll never know the danger of life on the range, coyotes and red men howling for your head on the other side of the campfire. "Once you have the hair back," he says, "you can tell the story."

Epilogue

Naming Names
An Afternoon at the Hair Club Headquarters in Boca Raton

Sy Sperling wants to show me his breathing membrane, the latest, most up-to-date hair replacement technology available. A thin piece of gas-permeable polyurethane that can remain on the scalp for four to six weeks at a time and seems to sprout hair just like a human head, it is the pride and joy of his Hair Club for Men. Though he's happy to tell me all about it, and to send me a videotape of the latest Hair Club infomercial, he really thinks I should see it in person, at the Hair Club headquarters. Of course, I could just as easily have gone to one of the Hair Club branches here in New York to see this remarkable breathing membrane, but it's clear that Sy is really a ringmaster at heart, a Catskill's *tumler* who wandered out of the Borscht Belt and now owns a national company that manages seventy to eighty million dollars a year in sales. His booming enthusiasm, made more boisterous by the frequency of his Bronx "aw"—as in Hair Club "*faw*" Men—is infectious, though, and within a couple of weeks I'm on a plane to Boca Raton, home of the Hair

Club headquarters and the Hair Club president, Sy Sperling, who is also, by the way, a client.

Before I see Sy I have plans for breakfast with a friend, Beatrice Greenberg, who is in the midst of planning her ninety-second birthday party but has time for a quick bite anyway. Bea lives in one of those places that make Florida what it is, a retirement community with specially designed quarters for all the different stages of old age, a shining square pool, grape arbors, and palm trees that look like they've been planted by Dr. Seuss. Inside the cool lobby, which is scattered with groups of huge, ripely cushioned chairs, are the telltale signs of managed recreation: posted notices of aqua exercise and movie times, a reminder that the bus for the conservative synagogue leaves an hour and a half earlier than the bus for the reform synagogue. On our way to the dining room, I ask Bea if she sits in these cushy chairs in the afternoon and talks with her friends. She stares at me as if I'm suggesting nude sunbathing in the parking lot. "I wouldn't talk to the people who sit here," she says, dismissing all of them with her hand. "My crowd meets in the bar."

When we get to the dining room, our seats have been rotated to the left of Bea's original choice, and she's a little annoyed. There's a busybody at our table whose husband is nice but who is always asking questions that Bea is not inclined to answer. Probably she moved our seats, though she doesn't respond when Bea asks if she did. To everyone who will stop to listen, Bea introduces me. "This is my friend Diane," she says. "She's here to interview some bigwig for her book." If they don't seem to register the significance of what she's said, she speaks a little slower, a little louder. "She's writing a book!" she shouts. "It's already been accepted!" Besides the busybody and her husband, there's a man named Bill at our table, too. He's brought Bea a half a banana this morning, and seems like a friend, so I tell him I'm in Boca Raton to interview Sy Sperling, the Hair Club guy. Everyone at the table nods politely, but uncertainly, so I follow Bea's example and try a little harder, slower, and louder. "He makes hair replacements—toupees?" Suddenly, everyone's smiling. They know toupees.

"Maybe you can help me," I say. "Did you ever know anyone who wore a toupee?" I've already spotted a guy whose hair is not his own on the other side of the dining room, and I'm hoping someone else has, too, but I'm getting blank stares again. The busybody looks confused. Bea grabs my arm and leans in close. "Listen, dear," she says confidentially, so I think maybe I've touched a nerve and the busybody's husband is wearing hair that is not his own. "All the men I knew either had *two* hairs on their heads, or *no* hairs on their heads." She turns back to her plate and slowly wraps Bill's half a banana in a napkin and puts it in her purse.

Toupee might be an okay word for a visit with Bea and her friends, but it's not acceptable at Hair Club headquarters, where the success of the breathing membrane depends on its *not* being mistaken for any form of outmoded "piece." Sy stands well over six feet tall, and though he is lean, his voice seems propelled by a deep diaphragm. "When you think of *toupee*," he lectures, "you think of the bad rugs out there—

the guys who look like they have a bird's nest on their heads. No one in the Baby Boom generation wants to be a toupee-wearer!" I have finally made it to Sy's, the Hair Club inner sanctum, and I am meeting with a gleeful Sy and his sober straight man, Mike Smith, the Hair Club's executive marketing director who is, of course, also a client. "When was the last time you saw *toupee* advertised?" Sy wants to know, really. "I invented the word 'system,' " he says proudly. This is one of his biggest contributions to the industry, the creation of a respectable, scientific vocabulary for hair replacement—no more embarrassingly foppish faux French. "System" is universal. "It's like Vaseline—it's become generic."

Not all Hair Club clients wear the breathing membrane. Some, maybe most, wear hand-tied, mesh-based systems, customized to match their hair growth pattern. But like the mesh system, the breathing membrane is polyfused to a wearer's head in a process whose name is more important than the underlying technology. "We don't stick it to the head," says Sy carefully, "we *polyfuse* it." I ask if he means they *glue* it, and he says no, it's not glued—it's *polyfused*. "It's painted, and it sticks," I say, pointing out the obvious similarities. But Sy sees where I'm headed. Yes, he agrees, but it's "not really glue." He's going to stick to his guns on this one. We settle on a compromise: polyfusion uses a "medical adhesive that's skin compatible." Then Sy offers a lesson in linguistic precision and market motivation. "There is a relationship to a wig, to a toupee, to a glue, but if we said, 'Come on in and buy a wig that's glued to your head,' nobody would ever come in." There are "primitive" and "barbaric" companies that would glue something to your head, Sy admits, but the Hair Club has their own "R & D"—research and development—department, which works hard to develop safe, simple, and palatable techniques like polyfusion, which, by the way, is a trademarked name.

Sy wasn't always the savvy, together guy he is now. In fact, the impetus to current success came in those years in his midtwenties when he was divorced, overweight, and combing his hair over into what he now laughingly calls a "retread." He lived, then, in suburban retreat with his sister Rosalie and her family in Deer Park, Long Island, avoiding social situations and a good long look in the mirror. His sister would tease him about his comb-over—"look at your part, it's by your ear!"—but young Sy couldn't face his situation and look for alternatives. Finally, Rosalie pointed out that he was always home on Saturday nights, and Sy sought help. He got a weave at one of the first black hair weaving salons in New York, Diane's Hairweaving, started hitting the singles scene, and found himself a career. "I lost weight," he remembers. "I bought new clothing, I went to Grossinger's . . . I got a whole bunch of phone numbers. The hair made a world of difference for me. I was a totally different guy. . . . It made me the person I wanted to be." Better than Prozac.

With the help of Walter Tucciarone, a member of the famous Tucciarone hair-processing family of New York, Sy and his brother, Jay Sperling, began a hair-weaving business. After a couple of false starts—one of Sy's early weaves wasn't done properly, and had to be cut out by his brother-in-law—Sy, Walter, and Jay developed a strong but light nylon base for the additional hair, and called it "The Tucci Original" after Walter, the "mad scientist" of the group. Even then, Sy was adamant: no toupees, no hairpieces. The Tucci Original was definitely a system, a way of life. Over time, the Sperling brothers parted company with Walter, who wrongly imagined he didn't need their marketing energies for his inventions. And a few years later, in 1973, Jay and Sy split up their partnership as well. Though it was almost ten years later that the Hair Club for Men began the television campaign that would broadcast Sy's before-and-after pictures across the country and make the Hair Club at home in ninety cities nationwide, the fraternal break is still a sore point.

Sy remembers doing his brother's hair at one point, and his sister-in-law calling and screaming at him because she hated it. "She didn't appreciate it," he says. "She was very critical." Now, his brother goes elsewhere for his systems. When I ask Sy how it looks, he shrugs and smiles with wicked indifference. "It probably could look better," he says. Still, Sy is wistful when he speculates about brotherly partnerships that survive. He thinks his brother, who is now in the home improvement business, probably still resents his success, though he doesn't show it anymore. Sy tries to be generous. His best memory from his early schooling at a Bronx yeshiva is the story of Joseph, who did not turn away his brothers when he became ruler of Egypt and they came looking for food. For a moment, Sy thinks about going to temple on Yom Kippur, the Jewish day of atonement. "A sin against your fellow man *isn't* forgivable," he says quietly. "A sin against God *is.*"

∞

The Hair Club headquarters sit unobtrusively near the top of a nondescript Boca Raton office building, at the edge of a wide boulevard lined with fuzzy palms and other nondescript office buildings. Inside, there is neither campy décor nor corporate pretension. For all their furious energy, the Hair Club offices have a distinctly mellow atmosphere: the so-called boardroom has a table and a few chairs, but Mike Smith shrugs when he sees them—they're not permanent, and the room's not even finished, and besides, there isn't really a "board." He's proud of the phone center, though, with twenty-five operators fielding calls from clients all over the country, and of the busy shipping room where hair replacement systems arrive from the Hair Club's factory in China, are sorted into cardboard boxes, and then shipped to the proper branch office. His own office is a neat, calm place with floor-to-ceiling tinted windows that look out on a soothing vista of grass, palm, and Florida road. But everything changes when Sy arrives. The even atmosphere is suddenly charged and jovial. Sy greets everyone before they greet him, usually with a nickname, a joke, or a cuff on the shoulder. Now the office resembles, well, a club—Sy's the cool guy who holds it all together, the hub of the wheel. He says he only comes in for a couple of hours each day, but it's clear those hours are essential. The company recently moved to Boca Raton to be nearer to him—he was needed, he tells me proudly, not even bothering to feign frustration. "I'm like Colonel Sanders at this point," he explains. "I don't make the chicken, but I tell people how to eat it."

Despite the plain décor, there's a bawdy feel to this Hair Club headquarters. In part, it's the nature of the industry, since restoring men's hair also means restoring masculine prowess. The infomercials that Mike Smith produces have the unlikely but unmistakable feel of soft porn: sultry saxophones purr in the background while good-looking men comb their newly dressed hair, attended by sexy, loving women. Over and over, they exclaim, "God! This feels great! Oh, it feels *so* good!" In part, though, the bawdiness is an emanation of Sy's personality. He is gregarious and, at the same time, humbly pleased that he is no longer an overweight kid with thinning hair. "God misinterpreted my prayers," he says, waits a beat and then delivers the punch line: "Instead of getting *balled* I went *bald*!" Ask him, and he'll tell you all about the two hours he spends every day working out. He watches CNBC and the *Today* show while he's on the Stairmaster. When I ask if the sexy blonde in the infomercial who plays his trainer is, indeed, his trainer, he is embarrassed but pleased. Mike interjects with a not-so-subtle jab to Sy's left. "No, Sy has his own trainer at home."

Perhaps this is vaudeville after all. Sy and Mike play at and off each other like Laurel and Hardy, Gracie and George, or maybe, Ernie and Bert. Whenever Sy says, "to say the least," Mike echoes with "the very least," and they crack up. After a while, they're ready for everyone's favorite game: "Toupee or no toupee," with Sy as the resident expert and Mike as his trusty assistant. Sy hams it up almost every morning, playing toupee gossip by phone with various radio hosts, and he recently got in trouble for a particularly revealing Howard Stern session, when he must have named names that did not want to be named, though neither he nor Mike will say any more. Now Sy is careful to introduce the rules of the game: he's offering his opinion, he stresses, not listing Hair Club clients and trading secrets. "We can just give opinions," he says, as much for his own benefit as for the tape I am rolling. "If you ask us what we think, we can give opinions." Briefly, they're willing to speculate about how you know someone's wearing hair that isn't their own: maybe the color is bad, maybe there's a hard frontal hairline, or too much hair crowning an older face. This is essentially a hunting exercise, a test of visual acuity. Can they spot the deer camouflaged in the woods? Sy and Mike watch the horizon religiously, looking for clues, but they're not miffed when they're wrong. Instead, they're hopeful. Mike loves to tell the story of being fooled by a Hair Club client; it means they're doing a good job.

So here we go. We start slow. I name the names, Sy gives his opinion. Tim Allen, Tom Cruise, Nick Nolte—Sy thinks they all have their own hair. Whitney Houston wears a weave and Nicholas Cage is definitely wearing "a little do-ski" and "it's not that good, either." Chuck Norris, Sy offers when I'm stumped; and how about Paul Reiser? "That's not his hair?" I ask, and in the corner of my eye I see a signal pass from Mike to Sy. Sy hesitates now. "No, I think he's got something."

When I ask why someone doesn't hurry up and help Marv Albert, Sy holds up his hand. "Marv has already been helped." Mike shifts uneasily in his seat, but Sy continues to speculate. "He looks a thousand times better. . . . I'm not gonna tell you any more about that one, but I can tell you he looks a lot better. Marv got the drift, basically. He got tired of the public ridicule. He probably went to a great place." By now, Mike might as well be using the hook to pull Sy off stage. "I'll leave it at that," says Sy. Donald Trump doesn't come to the Hair Club, but Sy certainly wishes he would. "My opinion is he's got something," asserts Sy. "I'd like to see him become a Hair Club client. We did his father, or we do his father. . . . I'd like to give him a better style."

I try to get Sy and Mike to focus on Robert Redford and Dustin Hoffman, but they won't. I can't tell what that means, so I move on.

Everyone knows Ted Danson wears a system, because sometimes he doesn't. This annoys Sy. "You don't want that," he warns. When I mention that it's really no different than Sy himself showing his before and after photos, bald and with his system, he shakes his head. "That's just a photograph, though! That's me, but it's not me. . . . Like John Travolta in *Grease*, 'It was me, but it wasn't really me.' "

Now Mike is excited, because he noticed a bald spot in a *Men's Health* photograph of John Travolta, a bald spot he'd never noticed before. It's right in the back, the same place Mike's hair has been thinning for several years now, though he's become the Hair Club guinea pig for a new laser treatment that Sy thinks will actually stimulate hair growth, and his bald spot is filling in quite nicely. The status of Travolta's hair is the kind of thing Mike and Sy will watch with the ardor of baseball fans near the close of a tightly played season. If the bald spot disappears, they know Travolta's "done something" about it. Even if he doesn't become a member, he'll have joined the club.

A Last Word About Hair Clubs, Past and Future

In the end, this is what I notice: more than our thoughts, habits, and desires, our hair longs for company. Even when it rejects one group and imagines it is unique, it is in reality cleaving to another. Those punk kids skateboarding through the park, their heads spiky and sprayed pink, have more in common with shag-cut cheerleaders and bristle-haired marines than they think. Sy's genius might not have been the scientific vocabulary he's lent the replacement industry. Instead, it is probably that four-letter word in the middle of the company logo. In this, Grouch Marx might have been wrong—most of us are happy to join the right club, even if it wants us as members.

For me, writing this book was a little like going to medical school and coming down with each new disease as it is covered in the textbook. I identified quickly and closely with each new problem that came along, chapter by chapter, and I joined each new group with a mixture of anguish and relief. Though it was hard to admit that I'd ignored the signs for so long, I gratefully accepted the belated wisdom of my fellow sufferers. Suddenly, I recognized the benefits of hot wax poured over the hairs that had crept stealthily past my bikini line. And it didn't take long to realize that a long, smooth, red-haired wig could cost less than a month's salary and might change my life completely. For fifty dollars, I reserved time at a salon in Harlem to begin the process of locking my hair—a funky, natural miracle cure for the kinky frizz that has plagued me most of my life. But when my stylist hurt her wrist I canceled my appointment. By then, I was talking to women about hair loss and locking seemed to call for undue pressure on potentially delicate follicles. How could I take that risk when the Rogaine tests seem so inconclusive and Propecia remains a man's drug?

We join the Elks and country clubs, sisterhoods, synagogues, and churches. Sometimes, we try to wear what our neighbors wear—those new capri pants, or that bulky barn jacket with the corduroy collar. And sometimes, when we can't get the look right, we plan for changes: a workout for our abs, a manicure, a nose job. But most of us don't volunteer for rhinoplasty. We jog so that our hips will seem smaller, and we go to salons to have our hair cut, colored, straightened, and permed. As a group, we spend billions every year trying to get our hair to look right. Why? A couple of years and all these pages later, I'm still not sure I know—why we spend so much money, why membership in the club is so necessary, why hair is so important, every day.

Perhaps it's because our hair begins inside of us, its roots invisible, and then grows outside. Some part of us must feel exposed by its journey, as if it carries secret truths from within and broadcasts them from the tops of our heads. Its health, well-being, and beauty reflect in some fundamental way our interior status—a periscopic reversal we can't control. Hence the association between sex and hair: it sprouts from the melted boundaries between inside and outside, secret and shared.

Lately, I've been covering my hair, with hats, bandanas, flowered scarves. I say it's because it's growing out—it's at that awkward stage between short and not-so-short—but that explanation only begs another question, really. The truth is that hair transitions are personal transitions, expressions of a deeper tumult—rough edges and breaking waves. I have written this book, my hair is getting longer, and the truth is, I'm not sure what happens next.

Selected Bibliography

The following bibliography is not an exhaustive catalogue of reference materials on hair; rather, it is intended to provide a list of the major materials I consulted in the writing of this book, and to gesture toward the sheer breadth of research possibilities.

Anderson, Jervis. *This Was Harlem: A Cultural Portrait, 1900–1950.* New York: Farrar, Straus & Giroux, 1982.

Angelou, Maya. *I Know Why the Caged Bird Sings.* New York: Random House, 1970.

"Are You Losing Too Much Hair?" *Glamour* (March 1998): 280.

Axtell, James. *The European and the Indian.* New York and Oxford: Oxford University Press, 1981.

———. *The Invasion Within: The Contest of Cultures in Colonial North America.* New York and Oxford: Oxford University Press, 1985.

———. *The School upon a Hill: Education and Society in Colonial New England.* New Haven: Yale University Press, 1974.

Bailey, Jeff. "The Comb-Over Loses Out in Battle Against Hair Loss." *Wall Street Journal* (September 29, 1998): 1.

Baker, T. Lindsay, ed. *WPA Oklahoma Slave Narratives*. Norman, OK: University of Oklahoma, 1996.

Banner, Lois. *American Beauty*. New York: Knopf, 1983.

Beavan, Colin. "New Strategies to Save Your Scalp." *Esquire* 127:4 (April 1997): 108–9.

Benjamin, Harry. *The Trans-sexual Phenomenon*. New York: Warner Books, 1966.

Bouchier, David. "What I Don't Need: Mirrors and Hair Loss." *New York Times* (November 8, 1998): 21.

Boulware, Marcus Hanna. *Jive and Slang of Students in Negro Colleges*. Hampton, VA: Marcus Boulware, 1947.

Brownmiller, Susan. *Femininity*. New York: Linden Press/Simon & Schuster, 1984.

Brumberg, Joan Jacobs. *The Body Project: An Intimate History of American Girls*. New York: Random House, 1997.

Chevannes, Barry. *Rastafari: Roots and Ideology*. Syracuse, NY: Syracuse University Press, 1994.

Cooper, Wendy. *Hair: Sex, Society, Symbolism*. New York: Stein & Day, 1971.

Corson, Richard. *Fashions in Hair: The First Five Thousand Years*. London: Peter Owen, 1965.

Davis, Angela. *Angela Davis—An Autobiography*. New York: International Publishers, 1988.

Davis, John Staige, M.D. *Scalping Accidents*. Baltimore: Johns Hopkins Hopsital Reports, 1917.

Didion, Joan. *The White Album*. New York: Simon and Schuster, 1979.

DuCille, Ann. *Skin Trade*. Cambridge, MA: Harvard University Press, 1996.

Earle, Alice Morse. *Two Centuries of Costume in America, 1620–1820, Vol. I–II*. 1903.

Ellinson, Rabbi Getsel. *Woman and the Mitzvot: The Modest Way.* Trans. Raphael Blumberg. Jerusalem: Eliner Library, 1992.

Epstein, Louis M. *Sex Laws and Customs in Judaism.* New York: Bloch, 1948.

Farrell, James J. *The Spirit of the Sixties: The Making of Postwar Radicalism.* New York and London: Routledge, 1997.

Fass, Paula. *The Damned and the Beautiful: American Youth in the 1920s.* New York and Oxford: Oxford University Press, 1979.

Fitzgerald, F. Scott. *The Beautiful and Damned.* New York: Charles Scribner's Sons, 1922.

———. *Flappers and Philosophers.* New York: Charles Scribner's Sons, 1920.

Foster, Helen Bradley. *New Raiments of Self.* New York and Oxford: Oxford University Press, 1997.

Frazer, James. *The Golden Bough: A Study in Magic and Religion.* New York: MacMillan, 1926.

Gates, Henry Louis, Jr. *Colored People: A Memoir.* New York: Knopf, 1994.

Geraci, Ron. "A Little More on the Top." *Men's Health* 13, no. 7 (September 1998): 130–5.

Gunn, Fenja. *The Artificial Face: A History of Cosmetics.* London: Newton Abbot, David & Charles, 1973.

Haiken, Elizabeth. *Venus Envy: A History of Cosmetic Surgery.* Baltimore: Johns Hopkins University Press, 1997.

Haltunnen, Karen. *Confidence Men and Painted Women: A Study of Middle Class Culture in America, 1830–1870.* New Haven: Yale University Press, 1982.

Hanover, Larry. "Hair Replacement: What Works, What Doesn't." *FDA Consumer* 31, no. 3 (April 1997): 7–11.

Hemingway, Ernest. *The Garden of Eden.* New York: Charles Scribner's, 1986.

Herskovits, Melville. *The Myth of the Negro Past.* New York and London: Harper & Bros., 1941.

Herzog, Dan. *Poisoning the Minds of the Lower Orders.* Princeton, NJ: Princeton University Press, 1998.

Hill, Christopher. *Society and Puritanism in Pre-Revolutionary England.* New York: St. Martin's Press, 1997.

Hitzig, Gary S., M.D. *Why Be Bald? Help and Hope for Hair Loss.* New York: Avon, 1997.

Hodges, Graham R. and Alan Edward Brown, eds. *"Pretends to be Free:" Runaway Slave Advertisements from Colonial and Revolutionary New York and New Jersey.* New York: Garland, 1994.

Holden, William. *Anti-Puritan Satire, 1572–1642.* New Haven: Yale University Press, 1954.

Horn, Barbara Lee. *The Age of Hair: Evolution and Impact of Broadway's First Rock Musical.* Westport, CT: Greenwood Press, 1991.

Hurston, Zora Neale. *Dust Tracks on a Road: An Autobiography.* Philadelphia: Lippincott, 1942.

———. "Story in Harlem Slang." *American Mercury* (Spring 1942): 84–96.

"If Narcissus Managed a Mutual Fund." *Fortune* 134, no. 5 (September 9, 1996): 70.

Jacobs, Andrew. "His Debut as a Woman." *New York Times Magazine* 147, no. 48 (September 13, 1998):48.

Jezer, Marty. *Abbie Hoffman: American Rebel.* New Brunswick, NJ: Rutgers University Press, 1992.

Jones, Dylan. *Haircults: Fifty Years of Styles and Cuts.* New York: Thames & Hudson, 1990.

Jones, Jacqueline. *Labor of Love, Labor of Sorrow: Black Women, Work and the Family, from Slavery to the Present.* New York: Basic Books, 1985.

Jones, Lisa. *Bulletproof Diva: Tales of Race, Sex and Hair.* New York: Anchor/Doubleday, 1994.

Kerber, Linda. *Women of the Republic: Intellect and Ideology in Revolutionary America.* Chapel Hill, NC: University of North Carolina/Institute of Early American History and Culture, 1980.

Levine, Lawrence. *Black Culture and Black Consciousness.* New York and London: Oxford University Press, 1977.

———. *Highbrow/Lowbrow: The Emergence of Cultural Hierarchy in America.* Cambridge, MA: Harvard University Press, 1988.

Lott, Eric. *Love and Theft: Blackface Minstrelsy and the American Working Class.* New York and London: Oxford University Press, 1993.

Major, Clarence, ed. *Juba to Jive: A Dictionary of African American Slang.* New York: Viking, 1970.

Martial. *Epigrams.* Trans. D. R. Shakleton Bailey. Cambridge, MA: Harvard University Press, 1993.

Marwicke, Arthur. *The Sixties.* New York and Oxford: Oxford University Press, 1998.

McCracken, Grant. *Big Hair: A Journey into the Transformation of Self.* New York: Overlook Press, 1996.

McCutcheon, Marc. *The Writer's Guide to Everyday Life from Prohibition Through World War Two.* Cincinnati: Writer's Digest Books, 1995.

Mencken, H. L. *In Defense of Women.* New York: Knopf, 1922.

Miller, Perry and Thomas H. Johnson, eds. *The Puritans,* Vol. II. New York and Cincinnati: American Book Company, 1938.

Miller, Timothy. *The Hippies and American Values.* Knoxville: University of Tennessee Press, 1991.

Morrow, Willie L. *Four Hundred Years without a Comb.* San Diego: Black Publishers of San Diego, 1973.

Muller, Richard W. *Baldness: Its Causes, Its Teatment and Its Prevention.* New York: Dutton, 1918.

Nessler, Charles. *The Story of Hair: Its Purposes and Preservation.* New York: Boni & Liveright, 1928.

Norwood, O'Tar. *Hair Transplant Surgery.* Springfield, IL: Charles C. Thomas, 1973.

Noyes, Nicholas. "An Essay Against Periwigs," in John Demos, ed., *Remarkable Providences: Readings on Early American History.* Boston: Notheastern University Press, 1972.

Padgett, Martin Jr. "In Thickness and in Health." *Men's Health* 13 (January–February 1998): 64–5.

Parsons, Elsie Clews. *Folklore of the Sea Islands, South Carolina.* Cambridge, MA, and New York: American Folklore Society, 1923.

Peiss, Kathy. *Hope in a Jar: The Making of America's Beauty Culture.* New York: Metropolitan Books, 1998.

Powdermaker, Hortense. *After Freedom: A Cultural Study of the Deep South.* New York: Viking, 1939.

Prosser, Jay. *Second Skins: Body Narratives of Transsexualism.* New York: Columbia University Press, 1998.

Roche, Daniel. *The Culture of Clothing: Dress and Fashion in the Ancien Regime.* New York and Cambridge: Cambridge University Press, 1989.

Rooks, Noliwe. *Hair Raising: Beauty, Culture and African American Women.* New Brunswick, NJ: Rutgers University Press, 1996.

Rubens, Alfred. *A History of Jewish Costume.* New York: Funk & Wagnalls, 1967.

Rubin, Bonnie Miller. "Hair Today, Gone Tomorrow." *Good Housekeeping* 225, no. 1 (July 1997): 42.

Rutman, Darrett B. *Winthrop's Boston*. Chapel Hill, NC: University of North Carolina/Institute for Early American History and Culture, 1965.

Sandomir, Richard. *Bald Like Me: The Hair-Raising Adventures of Baldman*. New York: Collier Books, 1990.

Sasek, Lawrence A. *Images of English Puritanism*. Baton Rouge: Louisiana State University Press, 1989.

Severn, Bill. *The Long and the Short of It: Five Thousand Years of Fun and Fury over Hair*. New York: David McKay Co., 1971.

Shakur, Assata. *Assata: An Autobiography*. Wesport, CT: L. Hill, 1987.

Shange, Ntozake. *Nappy Edges*. New York: St. Martin's Press, 1978.

Shapiro, Marc B. "Another Example of Minhag America." *Judaism* 39 (Spring 1990): 148–154.

Sinclair, Rodney. "Fortnightly Review: Male Pattern Adrogenetic Alopecia." *British Medical Journal* 317 (September 26, 1998): 865–9.

Truefitt, H. P. *My Views on Baldness, Being a Treatise on the Hair and Skin*. London, 1863.

Underdown, David. *Revel, Riot and Rebellion*. Oxford: Clarendon Press, 1985.

Villarosa, Linda. "Remedies for Hair Loss." *New York Times* (October 20, 1998): 7.

White, Graham and Shane White. *Stylin': African American Expressive Culture from Its Beginnings to the Zoot Suit*. Ithaca, NY: Cornell University Press, 1998.

Wolfe, Tom. *Radical Chic and Mau-Mauing the Flak Catchers*. New York: Farrar, Straus & Giroux, 1970.

Wood, Gordon S. *The Creation of the American Republic, 1776–1787.* Chapel Hill, NC: University of North Carolina/Institute for Early American History and Culture, 1967.

Woodforde, John. *The History of Vanity.* New York: St. Martin's Press, 1992.

———. *The Strange Story of False Hair.* London: Routledge and K. Paul, 1971.

Ziff, Larzer. *Puritanism in America: New Culture in a New World.* New York: Viking, 1973.